a-z of professional ethics

professional keywords

Every field of practice has its own methods, terminology, conceptual debates and landmark publications. The *Professional Keywords* series expertly structures this material into easy-reference A to Z format. Focusing on the ideas and themes that shape the field, and informed by the latest research, these books are designed both to guide the student reader and to refresh practitioners' thinking and understanding.

Available now

Mark Doel and Timothy B. Kelly: *A–Z of Groups & Groupwork*
Jon Glasby and Helen Dickinson: *A–Z of Inter-agency Working*
Richard Hugman: *A–Z of Professional Ethics*
Glenn Laverack: *A–Z of Health Promotion*
Neil McKeganey: *A–Z of Addiction and Substance Misuse*
Steve Nolan and Margaret Holloway: *A–Z of Spirituality*
Marian Roberts: *A–Z of Mediation*

Available soon

Jane Dalrymple: *A–Z of Advocacy*
David Shemmings, Yvonne Shemmings and David Wilkins:
    A–Z of Attachment Theory
Jeffrey Longhofer: *A–Z of Psychodynamic Practice*
David Garnett: *A–Z of Housing*
Fiona Timmins: *A–Z of Reflective Practice*

a-z of
professional ethics

Richard Hugman

palgrave
macmillan

First published 2014 by
PALGRAVE MACMILLAN

Palgrave Macmillan in the UK is an imprint of Macmillan Publishers Limited, registered in England, company number 785998, of Houndmills, Basingstoke, Hampshire RG21 6XS.

Palgrave Macmillan in the US is a division of St Martin's Press LLC, 175 Fifth Avenue, New York, NY 10010.

Palgrave Macmillan is the global academic imprint of the above companies and has companies and representatives throughout the world.

Palgrave® and Macmillan® are registered trademarks in the United States, the United Kingdom, Europe and other countries

ISBN: 978–0–230–33722–0

This book is printed on paper suitable for recycling and made from fully managed and sustained forest sources. Logging, pulping and manufacturing processes are expected to conform to the environmental regulations of the country of origin.

A catalogue record for this book is available from the British Library.

A catalog record for this book is available from the Library of Congress.

Printed in China

Dedicated to all my students

contents

acknowledgements

My thinking on the ideas presented in this book has taken shape over many years of practice, teaching and research. In that sense, it has been influenced by too many people to remember each by name here. Most especially, the students whom I have taught and with whom I have debated the subject of professional ethics have in turn taught me a great deal. While selecting particular individuals is a very difficult task, it is easier and a great pleasure to acknowledge the shared conversations with my doctoral students who have pushed me to clarify my thinking on ethics, values and related matters as much as I have theirs. These are (in alphabetical order) Birgitta Al-Issa, Loret Bartos, Rebecca Eckert, Mim Fox, Sacha Kendall, Shannon McDermott, Therese Milham, Nguyen Thi Thai Lan and David Palmer. I also have a huge debt to the ongoing influence of colleagues spread more widely afield, notably Laura Acotto, John Ang, Sarah Banks, Wendy Bowles, Elaine Congress, Mel Gray, Arne Grønningsaetter, David N. Jones, Donna McAuliffe, Maria Moritz, Salome Namicheishvili, Rory Truell.

As ever, the team at Palgrave Macmillan has been wonderful, with advice, support and patience – Catherine Gray, Katie Rauwerda, India Annette-Woodgate and Cecily Wilson. I am grateful to them for this.

And, as ever, anything missing, mistaken or contentious is entirely my own responsibility.

how to use this book

This book offers an account of the many ethical concepts that inform practice in what I have chosen to call the people professions (for reasons I explain further in the book's introduction). It is structured alphabetically into sections, where each addresses a single topic, be that *autonomy, responsibility, welfare* and so on. These topics are of different types, in the sense that some may be considered principles (i.e., the basis for a belief or way of thinking), while others provide broader conceptual tools for thinking about the moral aspects of the social world. However, together they are intended to provide students and professionals tools to engage in conscious reflection on their moral values. Each entry has been chosen because I believe it to have a key contribution to make to professional ethical debate. I discuss the rationale I used for choosing the 70 plus 'keywords' that follow in the book's introduction.

In writing the book, I have assumed that you will be using it as a resource, to examine particular ideas that have arisen in practice or study. The book's alphabetical structure means that it is designed to be dipped into according to interest and need rather than read from beginning to end. Each topic is therefore presented as a self-contained discussion, although there are many links between them (more on this is discussed later).

If you are new to the field of professional ethics – perhaps because you are taking a class on the subject for the first time and have been recommended this book to help your studies – you might find the entries on *values, competence* and *codes of ethics* particularly useful starting points. Alternatively, you might want to start with an idea that has a particular resonance for you (such as *compassion* or *respect*) or one that you feel a need to explore further (such as *confidentiality, justice* or *power*).

Many of the ideas that are presented and discussed in this book relate to each other. To allow you to pursue particular ideas and themes and aid connections between the different topics under discussion, several signposts are provided:

1. Each topic is listed in the contents.
2. Under the heading for each entry, there is a list of other topics that may be of potential interest. In effect, these are suggestions for what you might be interested to read next.
3. Within the text of every entry, I have italicized words that have entries of their own elsewhere in the book. For example, *integrity* is a *virtue* and both these terms have entries in the book. In each case, where the other term appears, it is in italics on the first occasion it appears. For consistency and clarity of meaning, at the point where such links are made, variations on such terms are also displayed, as in virtue, virtues and virtuous, compassion and compassionate, truth and truthfulness and trust and trustworthiness. Where some concepts are known by more than one word or term, cross referencing is clearly stated. For example, the reader looking for *African/Black ethics* is directed to the discussions of *ma'at, ubuntu* and *indigenous ethics*, the heading of *informed consent* will direct you to *consent* and so on.
4. Last but not the least, the book's index offers a more detailed map of its coverage. Do not forget to use this to supplement to the book's A to Z structure as not all the ideas contained within these pages could have entries in their own right. For example, I have located the key philosophers under the relevant entries and you will be able to locate them via the book's index. For example, Kant is discussed within the wider topic of *deontology*, Mill in relation to *utilitarianism*, Aristotle on 'virtue' and Plato regarding 'justice'. (Only Confucius is specifically accorded a distinct section, for reasons that are made plain there.)

Readers who are particularly interested to learn more about these thinkers and the legacy of their influences could consult histories of philosophy (such as MacIntyre, 1998) or an introductory text on ethical theory (such as Hinman, 2008). To assist with this, each entry concludes with suggestions for further reading for anyone who wishes to pursue particular points in greater depth.

Another widespread feature of the professional field is the tendency for each profession to engage with its own literature, often missing the ways in which other professions are thinking about the same issues, with potential insights to share. Books and journals continue to address tightly defined markets. On the basis of a review of volumes since 2000, even the prominent *Journal of Interprofessional Care* carries relatively few articles that address interprofessional thinking about ethics as a primary focus (see Clark *et al.*, 2007; Irvine *et al.*, 2002, for notable exceptions). Thus, with a view to contributing to greater interprofessional awareness and learning, I have included a range of professional sources in a dedicated 'further reading' section at the end of the book. These suggestions are necessarily indicative, not definitive. They include both generic and profession-specific publications.

introduction

In recent years there has been a considerable growth of interest in the field of ethics in what may be termed the 'caring', 'helping' or 'people' professions. Across all these professions, the ethical dimension of practice has come to be seen as one of the crucial dimensions of professionalism. At the same time, busy practitioners often face the need to understand the ethical aspects of their work. Those studying to become members of these professions also need to learn about the ethical dimensions of the skills and knowledge they are developing. Yet access to straightforward descriptions and discussions of the core principles and concepts involved is not always easy. This book provides a tool for everyone involved in such professions, at whatever stage in their career, to engage in a more informed consideration of the ethics of practice. How do we understand what is 'good' and 'right' in professional practice? This is the key question for everyone concerned with the professions and it is becoming more pressing in the face of the increasingly complex technologies and systems through which professional services are provided. In writing this book, I hope to provide an accessible introduction to the ideas that comprise professional ethics in the contemporary world, so that colleagues, students and others can find appropriate ways of answering this question.

What do we mean by ethics?

Ethics is often regarded as a matter of the rules of conduct in professional life. While it is certainly the case that such rules form a part of the field of ethics, it is important to recognize that ethics is much more than this. Although concerns with specific statements about conduct follow from ethical discussion, the main purpose of ethics is to have such a discussion in the first place. In this sense, ethics can be seen as 'the conscious reflection on our moral beliefs' (Hinman, 2012, p. 5). If ethics is understood in this way, it becomes clear that in order to engage with this aspect of professionalism practitioners need to develop an informed vocabulary.

In many situations, practitioners, students preparing for practice and those outside the professions, especially service users, rely on the formal statements about ethics that are made by the professional associations. Indeed, it is unthinkable in the modern world that a professional association would not have a code of ethics or a similar statement or document that could be used to determine whether a particular action is good or right, or otherwise. However, despite the obvious value of such documents, there remains the challenging task of applying formal statements to the messy nature of practice in the real world. Everyday life does not always provide distinct, clearly defined problems or issues to be resolved. While in many circumstances professionals use their own well-developed moral sense as the basis for decision making, there are also many situations in which choices are not necessarily clear-cut. It is in these sorts of situations that the capacity to address ethics in a conscious and deliberate way becomes necessary. (In the event that a practitioner's moral sense is not well developed, so that others find a reason to complain about someone's actions, codes of ethics do indeed function as rules or laws. This point is dealt with in this book in the section *codes of ethics*.)

So in this book, I approach the subject of ethics as something that all members of the professions should be engaged in. Many discussions of ethics in professional life concentrate on particular issues, or discuss concepts in greater depth. While such approaches are necessary, there is also a need to look at the core ethical ideas in a way that is accessible to practitioners, students and others. The point is that practitioners, students and others who are concerned with understanding professional ethics should not be expected to turn themselves into moral philosophers but rather be equipped to play an active role in the discussions and debates about what is good and right in their own particular discipline as well as in professional life more generally. As I observe throughout this book, questions with which ethics deals are too important to be left to experts alone, even though particular ethical expertise may be valuable in particular instances in helping to resolve challenges and dilemmas. In sum, the ultimate point of ethics lies in their application or effect. Therefore, in order to be able to contribute actively to this important aspect of professional life, every member, student or interested 'layperson' will gain from greater attention to the meaning of particular ethical ideas, concepts and terms.

Who is the book intended for?
In the selection and presentation of the 'keywords' discussed in this book, I have concentrated on those professions most often seen in terms of 'caring', 'helping' or 'people' professions (Bondi *et al.*, 2011; Hugman, 1991, 2005). This understanding of professions is used to refer to those occupations that in some sense can be said to have the 'person' of those for whom they provide services as the focus of their attention. These are the professions whose work directly affects people physically, mentally and psychologically, emotionally, spiritually or in terms of people's relationships. This includes the range of professions working in education, health, human services and social welfare. The primary audience for this book, therefore, includes audiologists, community workers, dieticians, medical practitioners, ministers of religion, nurses, occupational therapists, physiotherapists, psychologists, social workers, teachers and youth workers – and more besides. I have selected illustrations and explanations to ground the discussion in the everyday world of these groups. More widely, other professions such as lawyers, architects, accountants and others may find some of the ideas presented here to be useful, even though they are not the primary audience. They, too, are usually engaged with people in the provision of their services, even if the content of their work is not focused on the 'person' in the same way.

Ascribing notions such as *care* or 'helping' to professions is both descriptive and evaluative. Descriptively, these ideas refer to the way in which knowledgeable and skilled tasks or functions are performed by practitioners with the intention of promoting the well-being of the person, group or community who receives a service. The evaluative meaning of these ideas points to the expectation that members of these professions demonstrate a moral commitment to such well-being. As Koehn (1994) argues, the heart of ethics in the profession is that the main focus of practice is reflected in the value that each profession seeks to promote. For allied health, medicine and nursing, it is the value of 'health'. For teachers it is the value of 'education'. For social workers, youth workers and others in the human services, the central value is that of 'social well-being'. Other such examples will no doubt occur to the reader. This understanding that professionalism is, at its centre, an ethical enterprise, provides a workable device to address these professions together, rather than focusing on the differences and variations between them that is so often emphasized. It is on these grounds that I am able to refer mostly to these professions as a whole, rather than specifically, in the discussion that follows.

There are long-standing debates about the best term to use to describe the particular group of professionals I am writing for in this book. My own previous usage has been 'caring professions', and I have argued for a very precise meaning of 'care' (Hugman, 1991, 1998, 2005). However, this is contested, as others consider these professions often to be employed in activities other than caring, at least in the popular sense of the word. For example, they may perform a 'controlling' role in areas such as criminal justice, child protection and so on. The idea of 'helping' may be contested for similar reasons. So, for clarity, throughout this book I have used the term 'people' professions, with a view to emphasize their common focus on working with the public, whether directly in services for adults, children, families, groups or communities, or indirectly in management, policy or research roles (compare with Bondi *et al.*, 2011).

One important aspect of professional work that is not routinely shared is the terminology used concerning those people who receive services. The different professions variously refer to clients, patients, pupils and so on, according to the nature of the particular profession, its institutional basis of practice or its social and cultural milieu. As the discussion contained in this book looks at ethical concepts and ideas across a range of these professions, the more generic term of 'service user' will be applied. While it is recognized some members of these professions may regard this as clumsy, or even lacking precision, it serves the purpose of describing the common relationship between professionals and those who receive or make use of their services. It also avoids pre-empting some of the ethical questions that are addressed here, for example, whether the receipt of such services creates a hierarchical social relationship between service users and service providers.

Is there 'a' professional ethics?

If ethics is about conscious reflection on moral values, then professional ethics quite simply is the application of this process to the professions. Indeed, over many decades, the professions have become more aware of and responsive to the need for this critical thinking to occur. In many instances, this has happened separately for each professional, yet it is not only particular aspects of terminology such as the way in which we talk about service users that are specific to each caring profession, but also the detailed ethical literature. Each profession tends to discuss ethical concepts and questions separately from the other professions. While there has been some attention paid to interdisciplinary or multidisciplinary aspects of professional ethics (Hugman, 2005; Loewy and Loewy, 2004; Morrison, 2009), for the most part the field of professional ethics is a wide range of literature ranging across the various professions.

Yet the underlying foundation in moral philosophy of the ethics of each particular profession draws from a common stock of concerns. For this reason, at the applied level, I think that there are many helpful comparisons to be made. These can be seen clearly, for example, between the ethics of biomedical and health practices and those of what might be termed the 'social professions' (see Beauchamp and Childress, 2008, on the former and Banks, 2004, on the latter). They all address the implications of the same range of ideas as the basis of applied ethical statements. These include, particularly, the ethics of consequences, duties and virtues. Increasingly they may also include new developments in ethical theory, such as a concern with emotion, relationship, care, the environment, political discourse and so on (Hugman, 2005).

The major ideas that can be found across the caring professions are those that predominate wider ethical discussions. A brief review of codes of ethics and of the leading literature in each discipline reveals a particular concern with consequences, duties and virtues as ways of thinking about what is good and right in professional practice (Banks, 2006; Beauchamp and Childress, 2008; Carr, 2000; Fry and Johnstone, 2002; Fry *et al.*, 2010; Loewy and Loewy, 2004; Sercombe, 2010; Strike and Soltis, 2004; Tschudin, 2003). As such there are frequent points of direct comparison, even in many instances of strong similarities in the issues that are debated and the approaches taken.

Another feature of professional ethics, especially formal state-ments such as code of ethics, is the tendency for Western philo-sophical traditions to dominate. In particular, ideas from ancient Greece (notably those of Socrates, Plato and Aristotle) have set the foundation for much modern ethical thought. Subsequently these ideas were combined with Judaic and Christian values and then, more recently, have been approached in terms of rationality (removing the theological elements) (Bauman, 1993). In the proc-esses of colonialism and most recently globalization, Western ethics has come to set the terms of the debate worldwide and this is reflected in the documents of international professional bodies such as the World Medical Association (1964), the International Federation of Social Workers (2004), the International Council of Nurses (2006), the World Federation of Occupational Therapists (2006) and the International Union of Physiological Sciences (2008). Consequently, other traditions, such as those of Asia, Africa, or the Indigenous peoples of the Americas, Australasia and the Pacific, have tended to have had little influence. This is the case across the people professions (and other professions), although some recent scholarship has started to address this point (Clifford and Burke, 2009; Gabbard and Martin, 2010; Graham, 2000).

The commonality in ethical thinking between professions means that the concepts that are presented in this book may be read in terms of many forms of practice. It is actually difficult to see how they might actually apply only to one discipline, although the ways in which they may and should be applied differ in detail. The dominance of Western approaches and concepts is also common, but where ideas from other parts of the world are coming to be addressed in formal professional discussions, I have endeavoured to include these. Examples include the concepts of *ma'at* and *ubuntu* from Africa, as well as entries on *Indigenous (first nations) ethics* and *Confucian ethics (including filial piety)*. Beyond these specific sections, I also explicitly consider non-Western ideas where these are relevant to other topics. In this way, I hope the presentation of each concept will broaden the attention of the people professions towards diverse ethical traditions, enriching thinking on these issues, as well as better reflecting the diversity of backgrounds of both practitioners and service users.

The book's focus and framework

There are many ways in which discussions of professional ethics can be presented. One approach that is popular for practice issues is to focus on the details of particular applied questions – 'how should a nurse deal with this problem?' 'what are the issues facing a therapist here?' and 'is this the right way for a teacher to resolve this dilemma?'. Such discussions have great value, as they enable practitioners to identify with the real world aspects of the concepts that are being debated. However, they also emphasize the distinctiveness of each profession and obscure the commonalities. In contrast, a multidisciplinary approach to ethics permits insights and struggles to be shared across professional boundaries so that we can learn from each other. While the details certainly differ, many common problems faced by people professions have common bases and thinking about them is enhanced by considering different points of view. It is this inter-professional approach that I have used to inform in this book.

More philosophically oriented discussions might approach questions of professional practice in terms of particular theories. Examples would include discussions of duties (*deontology*), of consequences (such as *utilitarianism*) or of moral character (*virtues*). Others present arguments concerning the ways in which theories might be combined or work together, in what is known as 'ethical pluralism' (Hinman, 2012) or 'common morality' (Beauchamp and Childress, 2009). However, while these concepts are all considered in this book, the approach taken is to focus on distinct concepts. This is more the level at which most busy practitioners, students and others address ethical ideas to help in making sense of concrete practice concerns. So it is also the level at which a discussion of the kind presented here is able to make the same type of connections with practice. The book's underlying approach is pluralist, in that it draws on a wide range of ideas and does not seek to argue for one as paramount. You will find my justification for this in the section on *pluralism*.

Sellman (1996) argues for the notion of *moral fluency* as the main aim of professional ethics education. This is not only a matter of being aware of the implications of accepted norms but also to develop the capacity to think ethically for oneself, to make sense of options and to be able to ground practice in the deliberate exercise of moral choices. I do not claim to provide specific answers to ethical questions, challenges or dilemmas. What I offer here are accounts of the concepts that form the building blocks of ethical reflection and debate in the people professions. I do so with the hope of contributing to the moral fluency of the professions and through that helping to promote good practice.

a

African/Black ethics

SEE ALSO Indigenous ethics; ma'at; ubuntu

Writers such as Graham (2002) have argued that there is a distinctive Pan-African ethics that should be addressed by members of the people professions. However, the ethical ideas that together comprise this concept can be seen as distinct. Therefore, they are considered in separate sections of this book, under the terms *ma'at* and *ubuntu*. The section on *Indigenous ethics* is also of relevance to this topic. (Key texts are indicated in each of these sections.)

altruism

SEE ALSO beneficence; benevolence; virtue

In many cultural contexts, the idea that doing something for another person, for a group or even for an ideal or a cause, without the expectation of receiving anything in return, is considered to be a *virtue*. This is altruism.

The central moral quality of altruism lies in placing regard for others at the centre of one's actions, as opposed to consideration for one's self. For this reason, it can sometimes be considered as the personal capacity to be 'other-directed'. The altruistic person looks outwards from their own position and interests, basing their thoughts and actions on the interests of other people.

In describing a thought or an action as altruistic, it is also necessary to take into account whether it was engaged in freely. Acting in the interests of others may be coerced, either by circumstances or even (if perhaps rarely) by force. Under such conditions, such actions could not be considered as altruistic because their basis would lie in obedience, conformity, self-protection or some other reason or motivation. Understanding altruism in terms of other-directedness and freely chosen action raises a question about whether it is possible to separate a person's commitment to this value, or to beliefs or ideals that express it in some way, from any emotional, psychological or spiritual benefit that the person acting may gain as a result of her or his actions. This is the claim that altruism cannot really exist, because even if claiming to be other-directed the person who is acting may nevertheless gain a sense of satisfaction or pleasure from what they are doing. In other words, this criticism argues that people choose to do those things that they think are important and ultimately the underlying (or 'real') beneficiary will always be the person acting, because the outcome is that they 'feel good' or they see their own values being promoted. However, this seems unduly cynical, as this argument suggests that self-interest can be the only motivation for any act. While it may be the case that any act impacts on the person acting, and that such outcomes may be positive, this does not explain the choices that people make to act in ways that have clear, tangible costs of some kind, and where the consequent benefits for themselves are intangible and even apparently disproportionately small relative to the act involved.

One clear example of this is in the practice of donating blood. The primary purpose of collecting human blood is to provide transfusions for victims of accidents, people undergoing surgery and other life-saving procedures. Although there are countries where supplies of human blood are purchased, there are also many others where this is achieved through voluntary donations (such as Australia, New Zealand and the United Kingdom). In a significant study of this system, Titmuss (1971) argued that it constituted a public expression of altruism, in which people are in a 'gift relationship' with unknown others. While it may be the case that part of the motivation for donating blood without payment is in the emotional, psychological or spiritual benefit for the donor, it is also the case that the inconvenience and other aspects of the process deter some eligible donors (it takes time, it has to be done at designated clinics, it involves a minor medical procedure and so on). These represent quite tangible costs to the donor, compared with the more intangible benefits such as feeling that one has 'done the right thing'.

Members of the people professions may also choose to act in ways that may be considered altruistic. These can be in relatively minor ways, such as in undertaking tasks that are not a necessary require-ment of one's role (but for which one has the capacity) because a need is recognized and where not acting would not be considered as bad in the sense of being negligent or neglectful. A nurse might get a personal item for a patient who does not have family to do this, a teacher might spend time with a student who is having difficulty with their studies during a break time or a social worker make a domiciliary call to an older person who is isolated and worried when this could reasonably have been left to another day. On a larger scale, some entire career choices are altruistic. Examples include practitioners who choose to work in less glamorous or less well-paid parts of their profession or to work in parts of the world where conditions present significant challenges (such as situations of conflict, natural disaster and so on), where they could choose to do otherwise and such choices would be reasonable.

Simply choosing to work in a people profession itself is not necessarily altruistic. All these professions help people to meet their needs in a number of ways. Yet usually this is done for a fee or a salary, which is a tangible benefit. The practice of such professions becomes altruistic in circumstances where it meets the criteria of not seeking a tangible reward that might reasonably be sought and of being undertaken freely. In these conditions, it is possible for altruism to be seen in professional practice.

KEY TEXTS
- Glannon, W. and Ross, L.F. (2002) 'Are Doctors Altruistic?' *Journal of Medical Ethics*, 28 (2): pp. 68–69
- Steinberg, D. (2010) 'Altruism in Medicine: Its Definition, Nature, and Dilemmas', *Cambridge Quarterly of Healthcare Ethics*, 19 (2): pp. 249–257
- Straughair, C. (2012) 'Exploring Compassion: Implications for Contemporary Nursing. Part 1', *British Journal of Nursing*, 21 (3): pp. 160–164
- Titmuss, R. (1971) *The Gift Relationship* (London: George Allen & Unwin)

autonomy

SEE ALSO consent; deontology; freedom; human rights; liberalism; responsibility

How *free* is a service user to decide what help they will receive and how it will be provided? How free is a professional to make decisions about the way in which they will practise? These questions point to the important idea of autonomy, which is one of the central principles in modern Western ethics; it also underpins political democracy. However, there are several competing nuances to the idea of autonomy, each of which emphasizes different aspects and has different implications. This can make debates about autonomy complex and the term has a variety of detailed applied meanings.

Within Western philosophy, the idea of autonomy since the work of John Locke (1632–1704 CE) has tended to refer to the capacity of individuals to exercise moral discretion. Thus it is widely seen as a matter of each individual being as free as possible to make choices. Such freedom not only includes a lack of tangible coercion, but also whether people live with minimum constraints on the way in which they can decide what is good in life and are able to pursue such goods. For example, it is not only a matter of whether someone is literally forced to enter a particular profession (which may not happen often), but also how people's capacities to make a choice of career is affected by the way in which they are free to think about the values of different choices. This might be seen in weighing up the difference between a career that is focused on community service as opposed to another in which success is measured by having a high income. Such an understanding is the basis for the philosophy of *liberalism*, in which individual liberty is regarded as a primary value (because it enables preferred goods to be pursued). Yet this is not simply a mechanism that permits the maximum degree to which people can exercise choices, but goes to the centre of understanding 'what it is to be human.' Thus, liberalism sees the denial of autonomy as the negation of the core of humanity.

However, this does not mean that liberals regard autonomy as limitless. Locke's work refined the earlier ideas of Thomas Hobbes (1588–1679 CE), who had argued that society depends on an implicit agreement between people not to harm each other in the pursuit of preferences. In turn, this necessitates people accepting that there are limits not only to what can be achieved but also in what may be reasonably pursued in the first place. This idea is often called 'the social contract'.

The principle was further developed by Immanuel Kant (1724–1804 CE), who concluded that because human beings are rational and autonomous, we make our own moral laws. The model of ethical decision making that Kant developed is formal and empha-sizes that each person is her or his own individual ethicist: we decide for ourselves what are the best principles for evaluating choices between alternative courses of action. In this approach, the limits to the range of morally acceptable choices are more abstract, in that Kant proposes that a morally acceptable action must be based on principles that can be applied to every other person. That is, we cannot make claims to do something we would not allow others to do (an idea that is often rendered as 'do not do to others that which you would not wish them to do to you'). Thus, although the prac-tical outcome resembles Hobbes' ideas that morality holds society together, the way in which 'the good' is decided in this model is much more individualistic.

Nevertheless, whether it is Hobbes' or Kant's understanding that is accepted, it makes little sense to interpret the principle of autonomy as leading to a world in which people are all disconnected from each other and where each pursues their own preferences with no thought about other people. Rather, the core of this idea is the notion that to be human is to play an active role in our own lives. This involves being able to form thoughts, to experience emotions and the physical senses, to make choices within the finite nature of the world and to form relationships. These are aspects of what it is to be human that Sen (1983) and Nussbaum (2000) have called 'capabilities'. This does not concern individual physical or mental 'abilities', but rather refers to the way in which the social world is organized and whether people are enabled to live their lives in ways that they think are important. This view states that a good human life consists of what people have the possibility of doing rather than what they possess.

It should be noted that although this concept is based on liber-alism, it places relationships such as family, friendship, community and so on at the centre of a good life. So, for example, the criticism that the principle of autonomy is contrary to valuing family relation-ships, cultural traditions and so on is actually a reflection of the way in which particular interpretations of autonomy have become domi-nant in certain parts of Western societies. This is particularly impor-tant in debates between cultural perspectives. For example, some Asian and *African* views regard autonomy as a principle that reflects Western culture, along with that of *human rights* with which it is closely related. However, such an argument treats Western culture as homogenous (whereas autonomy is understood differently in varying parts of the West and between different communities, families and even individuals). Against such a view of autonomy, it should also be remembered that Western values include concepts such as selfishness. This can be considered as a 'vice', following the classic model of Aristotle (384–322 BCE) in which a vice is a negative extreme on either side of *virtue*: here selfishness is either a deficiency of regard for others or else an excess of regard for one's self. Thus the limit on autonomy is endemic in the social nature of human life.

Considering in this way, it becomes clearer that autonomy is not only about having as wide a range of actions as is possible, but also of having the capacity to take *responsibility* for one's actions. The morally autonomous person is not only able to exercise choice and pursue preferences but also to be accountable for the choices made and the actions that followed. Indeed, in making choice to pursue preferences we must each accept that our actions will have an impact on others, who then like ourselves have autonomy. Understood in this way, autonomy is not individualistic in reality, but is relational.

Partly because the modern forms of professionalism have been heavily influenced by Western societies, the ethics of the people professions tend to place great importance on the idea of autonomy. In medicine, Beauchamp and Childress (2009) take this as one of the four core ethical principles. They are concerned that in all aspects of medical practice there is a potential for significant change to be made to the bodies or minds of patients and so to impact on all areas of their lives. If patients are treated without giving their agreement, then their humanity is denied. From this, ideas such as *consent* to medical procedures have developed. As the objective of medicine is to restore people to as full a human life as possible, this is congruent with the view that autonomy is part of such a life. This gives medical practitioners, and other health professionals (Tschudin, 2003), a duty to respect the capacity that service users have for making decisions about their own lives. In some cases, this might even include a refusal or withdrawal of consent, which then prevents the practitioner from providing treatment.

Social work tends to talk in terms of self-determination, which is a related concept (Banks, 2012). This is often seen as a form of Kantian ethics, but as Banks notes in practice some limitations tend to be set on it. Law and policy, for example, may make some preferences difficult or impossible to achieve. It is also likely that in some situations that the choices one person might wish to make will have a detrimental effect on others. So in practice, social workers, like colleagues in the other people professions, find themselves having to prevent people from following certain courses of action. This can be seen in statutory fields, such as child protection, mental health and criminal justice. In this sense, Banks agrees with Beauchamp and Childress and others that autonomy, or principles based on it such as consent and self-determination, cannot be considered absolute.

KEY TEXTS

- Beauchamp, T.L. and Childress, J.F. (2009) *Principles of Biomedical Ethics*. 6th edn (New York: Oxford University Press), Chapter 4
- Bowles, W. *et al.* (2006) *Ethical Practice in Social Work* (St. Leonards: Allen & Unwin), Chapter 6
- Le Granse, M. *et al.* (2006) 'Promoting Autonomy of the Client with Persistent Mental Illness', *Occupational Therapy International*, 13 (3): pp. 142–159
- Scheyett, A. *et al.* (2009) 'Autonomy and the Use of Directive Intervention in the Treatment of Individuals with Serious Mental Illnesses', *Social Work in Mental Health*, 7 (4): pp. 283–306

b

beneficence

SEE ALSO altruism; benevolence; care; non-maleficence; responsibility; utilitarianism

As with *autonomy*, beneficence is one of the four principles claimed by Beauchamp and Childress (2009) as central to biomedical ethics (see also Tschudin, 2003). In its simplest form, the idea of beneficence refers to the promotion of the good of others. Thus it is connected to *altruism* and *benevolence*. However, it differs from them in that beneficence can be seen as the pursuit of outcomes promoting the good, rather than the attitude or disposition of the person acting. It is best expressed in the goal of 'seeking to do that which is good', defined as that which benefits the service user.

Although Beauchamp and Childress (2009, p. 198) argue that the principle of beneficence has a long history, for example, seeing it in ancient religious texts as well as in Hippocrates' teaching, most of the attention to it in ethics has been in recent times. In this context, it is seen as particularly applicable to those who have particular roles to play, such as members of the people professions. For professional practitioners, this principle turns acting for the benefit of the service user from a functional description into a moral requirement. It is a duty because acting for the benefit of service users is the reason the practitioner was trained, earns a fee or a salary, holds a particular standing in the community and so on (Koehn, 1994).

The way in which the principle of beneficence is enacted has several dimensions. First, it requires that the practitioner carefully attend to the balance between benefits and risks in a particular action. In this sense, 'taking care' should not be seen as identical to the 'ethics of care' (see *care, ethics of*), although it may be related in that it suggests using skills and knowledge in ways that are attentive and responsive to the service user. The key point is that when risks are greater than expected benefits, then the practitioner should find an alternative course of action. As Tschudin (2003, p. 64) notes, where the risks outweigh expected benefits, the principle of *non-maleficence* (or non-malfeasance: do no harm) should take priority.

Second, beneficence assumes that the benefits for the service user are at least as significant as any that the professional practitioner might gain. Where there is any conflict of interest, then those of the service user should be primary. Again, this is not the same as altruism or benevolence, as the practitioner can still reasonably benefit (e.g. an income). Nor does it require that the benefits achieved by service users and professionals must be of comparable types. Where the service users gain improved health, an education, resolution of family or community problems and so on, professionals earn a living, improve their expertise, teach students in their field, conduct research and so on. The point is that service users should not be put at risk, disadvantaged or even just inconvenienced for these goals to be pursued.

Third, beneficence can be understood as a type of *consequentialist* ethics. That is, judgments about what is good and right may be based on consequences or outcomes. However, because in most situations outcomes can be predicted but not guaranteed, such judgements depend on following the best available knowledge about what can be expected to occur rather than relying on what actually happens (see *rule utilitarianism*). This is where the principles of autonomy (by involving the service user in decision making as much as is possible) and non-maleficence (seeking to do no harm) helpfully balance the *responsibility* that beneficence requires.

KEY TEXTS

- Dodd, S.J. (2007) 'Identifying the Discomfort: An Examination of Ethical Issues Encountered by MSW Students during Field Placement', *Journal of Teaching in Social Work*, 27 (1): pp. 1–19
- Glannon, W. and Ross, L.F. (2002) 'Are Doctors Altruistic?' *Journal of Medical Ethics*, 28 (2): pp. 68–69
- Munyaradzi, M. (2012) 'Critical Reflections on the Principle of Beneficence in Medicine', *Pan-African Medical Journal*, 11, #29 [downloaded on 10/9/2012 from http://www.panafrican-med-journal.com/content/article/11/29/full]

- Oakes, C.E. (2011) 'In Their Best Interest: The Challenge of Balancing Autonomy and Beneficence in Clinical Practice with Older Adults', *Gerontology Special Interest Section Quarterly*, 25 (9): pp. 1–4

benevolence

SEE ALSO **altruism; beneficence; care; justice; virtue**

Although benevolence can be understood as a *virtue* in the ancient Greek sense, in his history of ethics MacIntyre (1998) attributes the modern development of the idea of benevolence to the British philosophers of the eighteenth century. In particular, David Hume (1711–1776 CE) is credited with asserting that benevolence is a primary human sentiment, one that promotes other virtues such as *justice*. In this sense, benevolence can be understood as an emotional or a psychological response to the humanity in others. So it is close to *altruism*; indeed it is usually the ground of that notion, but it is not the same.

A benevolent attitude can be seen as a basis for many of the ways that members of the people professions might aspire to act. In broad terms, it describes the intention that lies behind the pursuit of the value encapsulated in any given profession (Koehn, 1994). For the health professions this is health, for teaching it is education, for social work it is social welfare, for youth work it is the well-being of young people and so on. It must be noted that benevolence refers to a disposition to pursue these values, not the actual consequences of actions. So although it may be used to describe an action, this is because of what the action reveals about the moral intention of the practitioner.

One of the problems for the modern world with Hume's ideas is that he refers to benevolence as a 'sentiment'. Thus, it can now be heard as condescending or patronizing, as expressing a sense of social superiority on the part of the person who is said to be benevolent. In some fields, the idea of empathy has taken its place. Here empathy can be understood as the capacity to grasp the meaning of another person's life, from that person's point of view; in a helping relationship, this also requires the ability to communicate this understanding back to the other person. Although there may be an ethical dimension to the development and use of empathy (the practitioner ought to seek to develop this capacity), in itself it is a skill rather than a moral disposition. It focuses on the feelings and thoughts of the other person, not the person who has empathy. By contrast, benevolence can be regarded as a value orientation expressing the feelings and thoughts of the benevolent person.

Yet, despite the negative connotations of possible condescension, it is hard to consider the ethics of the people professions without the notion that these are practices based on a positive regard for the well-being of people. Of course, it is possible for any of these professions to be practised without a personal sense of benevolence, for example, in a situation where personal-care tasks are performed without any positive regard for the well-being of the person receiving them. However, in such a situation, it might be said that this is not good practice, or that it could be better, because of the ethical quality it embodies. (This point is developed in more detail in the section on the ethics of *care*.) For this reason, the notion of benevolence can assist in thinking about one's own orientation to the ethical goals of a profession and relationships with service users.

KEY TEXTS
- Ferguson, E., Farrell, K. and Lawrence, C. (2008) 'Blood Donation as an Act of Benevolence Rather Than Altruism', *Health Psychology*, 27 (3): pp. 27–36
- Mukherjee, G. and Samanta, A. (2005) 'Wheelchair Charity: A Useless Benevolence in Community-Based Rehabilitation', *Disability & Rehabilitation*, 27 (10): pp. 591–596

C

care (duty of)

SEE ALSO beneficence; care (ethics of); competence; consequences; duty; non-maleficence; responsibility

Increasingly in those countries where the connections between professional ethics and legal obligations are most highly developed, the notion of the duty of care has come to be of concern to practitioners. The basic concern is that practitioners take all reasonable steps to ensure their actions are to the benefit of service users (*beneficence*) and do not cause harm (*non-maleficence*).

The most important elements in considering duty of care are as follows: (1) does the practitioner have a *duty* towards a particular service uses of group of service users; (2) are there standards of what is 'reasonable' in terms of what should or could be known about the *consequences* of particular actions and (3) what scope for decision making does the practitioner have?

Banks (2012, p. 168) notes that professional roles have boundaries. The example that she uses is that of a person in serious financial need (who does not even have enough money for a cup of coffee). There is a difference, Banks argues between the moral responsibility that any person might feel on encountering someone in the street in such need, so that we might respond by giving them money from our own pocket or taking the person to a local café, and the duty on a social worker encountering the same person in her or his role in a district social work office, where procedures of assessment would need to be followed. Under such circumstances, for the social worker to provide money out of their own pocket would be beyond their duty (it would be *supererogatory*). This example can be extrapolated across the other people professions. The practitioner who declined to intervene because a particular need did not form part of their role would not be failing in their duty of care on those grounds alone.

Second, the idea of duty of care is based on an understanding of what is reasonable. The test that would normally be applied in this regard is that of the views of an ordinary but informed person, not just those who are members of particular professions. There are certain broad aspects on which it may be easy find agreement, such as in the example above of a person in acute financial need. However, there can be other situations where the line is less clear. For example, a medical practitioner or nurse who did not go to the aid of an older man who has collapsed on the floor of an airplane because they do not want to interrupt the movie they are watching might be seen as having made an unreasonable choice; similarly, a teacher who chooses not to interrupt the lunch break to assist a child who has hurt themselves even though the teacher is not 'on duty' will be seen to have acted unreasonably.

Third, a professional does not have a duty of care if the need with which they are confronted lies outside their sphere of *competence*. This is not always an easy matter to demarcate, as emotional, physical, psychological, social and spiritual needs often are not clearly separable. Nevertheless, each profession has its own broad areas of competence and it would be potentially detrimental for any practitioner to act beyond the limit of their knowledge and skills. There are times when this may need to be explained clearly to service users, who may not always be aware of the precise scope of each profession. The duty of the practitioner in this regard is to be clear about her or his own limitations.

In some countries, legal systems may blur the moral duty of care into legal obligations. Thus, for example, discussions by Reamer (2006) or Beauchamp and Childress (2009) in the context of the United States are slightly different than that of Tschudin (2003) or Banks (2012) in the United Kingdom. The legal frameworks are affected, in part, by cultural differences in notions of *responsibility* and the way in which these translate into expectations of redress. However, from an ethical perspective, the obligations that are embedded did the duty of care concern taking all reasonable actions; they do not imply a responsibility for success in particular situations. In other words, this duty is to practice to the best possible standards and not a guarantee of healing, learning, social well-being and so on.

KEY TEXTS

- Fulcher, L. and McGladdery, S. (2011) 'Re-examining Social Work Roles and Tasks with Foster Care', *Child & Youth Services*, 32 (10): pp. 19–38
- Hawkins, R. *et al.* (2011) 'Duty of Care and Autonomy: How Support Workers Managed the Tension between Protecting Service Users from Risk and Promoting their Independence in a Specialist Group Home', *Journal of Intellectual Disability Research*, 55 (9): pp. 873–884
- Richards, J.L. and Walker, R.N. (2011) 'Ninja Threats or Fantasy?' *Ethics & Behavior*, 21 (1): pp. 79–81

care (ethics of)

SEE ALSO **beneficence; benevolence; care (duty of); competence; emotion; feminist ethics; justice; responsibility**

In recent years, the arguments for an ethics of care have exerted an increasing impact on debates in the people professions. While it may seem tautological that these professions should have to attend to 'care' in their ethics, this is a particular approach that is not accepted by everyone.

The origins of the distinctive ethics of care lie in *feminist* theory, especially that of the late twentieth century (CE). Gilligan (1982) argues that ethical theory has tended historically to be dominated by masculine perspectives on the world, with the result that it tends to emphasize abstract rationality, duties and principles. While these may assist in thinking about what is good and right, the result has been the exclusion of considerations of social relationships as something to be valued in and for themselves. Therefore, a feminist perspective, one that asks what women's lives have to teach everyone, is seen as an important correction to this distortion.

Tronto (1993) identifies four aspects to the ethics of care: attentiveness, *responsibility*, *competence* and responsiveness (Table 1). Each of these matches a stage in caring as an act. These are aspects of relationships. For the ethics of care, sustaining and developing relationships is by itself a primary good. It also suggests a value orientation on the part of the person caring towards the well-being of the person who is cared-for. Nor is this a one-way process, it is a relationship in which the actions of the person cared-for are also part of the ethical consideration.

Element	Meaning	Matching 'phase' of caring
Attentiveness	Seeking to know and understand the person cared-for; moral disposition to recognize the need of others	Care about
Responsibility	Preparedness to act on what is attended to and then acting	Care for
Competence	Being equipped to respond to the person cared-for, in both skills and knowledge	Care giving
Responsiveness	Enabling and supporting the person cared-for to receive care and to have an active role in the relationship	Care receiving

TABLE 1 *The elements of the ethics of care*

In the people professions, the idea of the ethics of care has been most widely addressed from nursing. Johnstone (1994) is very critical of earlier arguments that nursing students should be taught 'less complex' ethics than, for example, medical students. This former view was based, largely, on the fact that the majority of nurses are women. Against this, Allmark (1995) questions whether the ethics of care actually has any value content. He asserts that it does not tell us what we should care for, or by what measure we may know that care has been achieved. In response, Bradshaw (1996) points out that care is not a commodity but rather must be seen as a combination of a moral disposition to the well-being of another person (comparable to *benevolence*) and a capacity to use the professional relationship as the basis for promoting that well-being. It is both a moral disposition and a skill, brought together in ongoing practice.

Jecker and Self (1991) raise the question of whether it is possible to separate the moral disposition and skill in caring, through a distinction between 'caring *about*' and 'caring *for*'. So, while the ideal situation may be that a practitioner will combine these two dimensions, insofar as practical caring is accomplished competently, this may not be a problem. The practitioner must practice competently, even if the service user is disliked or judged morally in some way (perhaps they can be seen as the cause of their own misfortune). The situations that should be avoided are in which the practitioner cares about but not for (in other words, feels benevolent towards the service user but does nothing) or does not care either about or for (and so rejects the claims of the service user altogether). Concerns about 'burn-out' are based on the idea that exposure to the demands of caring, without the person caring her or himself also being cared-for, can lead to the loss of benevolence that in turn reduces the capacity to be attentive, responsive or competent.

A further question about the ethics of care is the possibility that it may be contrary to the key notion of justice. This was debated particularly in the 1990s. Tronto's (1993) conclusion represents a developing consensus that it ought not to do be a matter of either/or. Of particular concern in this respect is the possibility that by valuing relationships, the sort of impartiality that is emphasized by other approaches to ethics is lost. Thus, it might be thought that the ethics of care may lead to practitioners favouring people with whom they have a basis for good connection, people like themselves, family and friends and so on. This concern is answered best by observing that partiality and particularity are not the same thing. Any practice has to be undertaken in a given context, one of particular relationships, between *this* practitioner and *this* service user in *these* circumstances (Hugman, 2005, p. 71).

Bauman (1993) also rejects the idea of care, but does so on the basis that it constitutes what could be called 'moral suffocation'. This is care understood as the imposition of a paternalistic view of the superiority of professional knowledge: 'the doctor knows best', 'do as the teacher says' and so on. However, there is a complex mix of issues here. Professional knowledge, by definition, is not possessed by those who do not have the training – that is a major reason people seek assistance from qualified professionals. Failure on the part of service users to act on professional advice is a significant problem in the success of professional helping. Yet Bauman may be partly correct insofar as practitioners must also engage with service users so that each understands the other as much as possible. The idea of responsiveness (see above) involves the interaction between the one caring and the person cared-for, in which both play an active role. From the perspective of the ethics of care, the good practitioner is the one who enables this to happen as much as is possible.

In summary, the ethics of care is not an abstract formula or set of principles, but should be understood as a framework that provides a basis for consideration of the relationships through which the practices of the people professions are achieved. It encourages practitioners to ask themselves important ethical questions, such as 'have I been attentive to this service user?'; 'have I taken responsibility to act to promote the well-being of the service user?'; 'have I used my skills and knowledge to my best ability (am I competent)?' and 'have I enabled the service user to be responsive to my practice and engaged with her or his responsiveness?'

KEY TEXTS

- Edwards, S.D. (2011) 'Is There a Distinctive Ethics of Care?' *Nursing Ethics*, 18 (2): pp. 184–191
- Orme, J. (2002) 'Social Work: Gender, Care and Justice', *British Journal of Social Work*, 32 (6): pp. 799–814
- Simpson, C. (2002) 'Hope and Feminist Care Ethics: What Is the Connection?' *Canadian Journal of Nursing Research*, 34 (2): pp. 81–94
- Tronto, J. (1998) 'An Ethic of Care', *Generations*, 22 (3): pp. 15–20
- Waghid, Y. and Smeyers, P. (2012) 'Reconsidering "Ubuntu": On the Educational Potential of a Particular Ethic of Care', *Educational Philosophy and Theory*, 44 (Supplement 2): pp. 6–20

codes of ethics

SEE ALSO consequentialism; deontology; pluralism; principles; principlism; responsibility; utilitarianism; virtue

In the modern world, it is difficult to think of a profession that does not possess a code of ethics. Indeed, some studies of professionalization take this to be one of the hallmarks of professionalism (Freidson, 2001). However, these vary in length and detail between different countries and between different professions. For example, some are short statements or affirmations of moral intent, while others provide extensive guidance on ethical principles and how these should be applied in various practice situations (Johnstone, 1994; Hugman, 2005; Beauchamp and Childress, 2009; Banks, 2012). So they can vary from a one-page 'oath', intended to be recited aloud by a newly qualified practitioner, to books that can be considered as 'rules' or 'laws' of good and right conduct.

Codes of ethics perform a number of functions. First, they enable a recognized professional group, such as a professional association or guild, to make clear statements to its own members and to those outside the profession about its values. A member of the profession, a member of another profession or a member of the wider society can all examine the code to see what is the moral basis of practice in this specific profession. Second, codes of ethics can be used to evaluate practice. They enable the question 'is this good practice for this profession?' to be addressed. When a practitioner is concerned to know how a particular action would be perceived, or someone finds fault with a practitioner's action, a code of ethics provides the benchmark against which judgements can be made. Depending on the legal system of a country, this function may provide the basis for redress by someone who is aggrieved about what they consider to be bad practice. Third, a code of ethics can make aspirational statements about what ought to be the case. Thus it can serve to promote improvements in practice.

Although a code of ethics is a single document, many are written from what can be understood as a *pluralist* or common morality approach to ethical theory (Beauchamp and Childress, 2009; Banks, 2012). That is, codes do not normally adopt one particular ethical theory (such as *deontology* or *utilitarianism*), but seek to combine these either by applying them differently to various aspects of practice, or by looking at the core principles that each approach shares with other approaches as the foundational ways of thinking about ethics. This sort of plurality can be seen in the ethical codes of allied health, medicine, nursing, psychology, social work, teaching and youth work. For example, all of these professions in many countries value respect for people as human beings, from which ideas such as *autonomy* and *human rights* are derived. At the same time, they also value *justice*, which has *consequential* elements. Similarly, some also make reference to professional *virtues* in the form of desirable qualities of a practitioner, such as *benevolence*. Indeed, the work of Beauchamp and Childress (2009), which had a major impact across all the biomedical and health professions and beyond, explicitly combines autonomy, *beneficence, non-maleficence* and justice in a 'common morality' model.

It is also important to distinguish between codes of ethics and codes of conduct or standards of practice. Statements about conduct may be included in a code of ethics, but this also will be in the context of explicit presentation of the moral bases for practice. Moreover, a code of ethics applies to all members of a profession. By contrast, a code of conduct is a descriptive document that does not rely on ethical argument as such. Perhaps more importantly, a code of conduct applies to people employed in a specific organization and may include members of many professions and other colleagues. Standards of practice apply across a profession, but these are documents that specify levels of knowledge and skill, and possibly ways that these ought to be applied. However, the 'ought' here is more a matter of technical performance and although reference may be made to a code of ethics, this is usually treated as something outside the statement of standards, as supporting ideas.

Codes of ethics have grown in importance alongside the growth of modern forms of the professions. They have become increasingly important in the people professions following atrocities in the conflicts of the twentieth century (CE). Not only medicine, but also nursing, teaching and social work were implicated in the events in Europe in the Holocaust (Johnstone, 1994). By emphasizing ethics as the basis of moral *responsibility*, it is intended that this might be avoided in the future. This background to the growth of attention to codes of ethics, as well as the abstract rationality with which many are written, reveals their origins in Western ethical thought. For this reason, in some other parts of the world, codes of ethics do not have the same significance, or else they are accepted as 'something that a profession has to have', without being integrated into thinking about practice. International organizations, such as the International Council of Nursing (2006), the International Federation of Social Workers/International Association of Schools of Social Work (2004), the International Union of Psychological Science (2008) and the World Medical Association (2006), have ethical documents that are used in some countries as codes of ethics.

In addition to using codes of ethics as rules or laws, it is also possible to regard them as frameworks for ethical engagement.

For the practitioner who is concerned to become more *'morally fluent'*, the code of ethics provides the basis for entering the ethical conversation of their profession. Whichever position is adopted, however, codes of ethics are an important tool for modern practice.

KEY TEXTS
- Banks, S. (2012) *Ethics and Values in Social Work*. 4th edn (Basingstoke: Palgrave Macmillan), Chapter 4
- Tschudin, V. (2003) *Ethics in Nursing: The Caring Relationship*. 3rd edn (Oxford: Butterworth-Heinemann), Chapter 5

community

SEE ALSO **autonomy; Indigenous ethics; ubuntu; values**

Values do not come from within people as isolated individuals, but as members of social groups. As individuals we hold beliefs and preferences through our relationships with other people. In that sense, our values come from our membership of communities. The idea of community is many dimensional: as many as 96 different interpretations have been identified by social scientists (Butcher *et al.*, 2007; Tesoriero, 2010). In broad terms, it can refer to shared culture and ethnicity, a neighbourhood or even shared membership of a profession. Such groups or networks are often held together by shared values. So it makes sense to talk about 'professional values': these are part of belonging to the same profession.

A sense of community is also a value by itself. That is, this is something that people regard as an aspect of living well. We may feel that things are right when we are able to share beliefs, ideas and values with others so that we experience a sense of belonging to a group. Maslow (1954) identified this as a basic human need. From this idea, it may be argued that an overly individualistic understanding of *autonomy* is implausible. It is not that we experience life simply as a community member with no sense of individuality, but rather that our individuality is formed and lived in the relationships and networks of our communities. In modern, highly complex societies, our individuality is formed as members of multiple communities, in which we may differ from other members of any one of those groups.

The value of community also figures strongly in *Indigenous* ethics and in the *African* concept of *ubuntu*. If, as these world-views emphasize, the identity of individuals can only be understood in terms of membership of communities, then belonging and shared values must be regarded as goods in themselves. In these ethical approaches, community is not simply a facet of the lives of individuals, but is primary, acting as the bedrock on which human lives are lived.

In practice, in whatever cultural context, this means that it is important to understand both one's own community memberships and those of service users. This can be experienced both in inter-disciplinary and multi-disciplinary work and also in working with people from other cultures and ethnicities. From a relational perspective, there is an ethical reason to attend to this dimension of human life, because unless we do so we may fail to address the humanity of those with whom we work, either as colleagues or as service users. One expression of this can be found in the concept of 'cultural competence'. However, this must not be reduced to a technical matter of skill and knowledge, but it is better understood as the development of an ethical orientation to the particularities of others as they regard the world from their own point of view (see *competence* in this volume).

KEY TEXTS
- Butcher, H. *et al.* (2007) *Critical Community Practice* (Bristol: Policy Press)
- Sercombe, H. (2010) *Youth Work Ethics* (London: Sage Publications)
- Waghid, Y. and Smeyers, P. (2012) 'Reconsidering "Ubuntu": On the Educational Potential of a Particular Ethic of Care', *Educational Philosophy and Theory*, 44 (Supplement 2): pp. 6–20

compassion

SEE ALSO care (ethics of); consequentialism; dignity; human rights

Compassion literally means 'feeling with' or 'feeling alongside' another person. This has the sense of recognizing the plight of another person and seeing this as something that evokes a feeling of common humanity. This is similar to the notion of attentiveness in the ethics of *care*. However, the idea raises some problems for ethics because not every plight experienced by another person can be expected to generate such feelings.

Nussbaum (2001, Part II) makes some helpful comments about compassion as an intelligent emotion. First, she notes that to regard a situation as a plight requires acceptance that it is significant. This does not relate to matters that can be seen as trivial or relatively minor: compassion is felt when we see that another person is facing a 'tragic predicament'. Moreover, we can agree that life would be more fulfilled without having to experience such a plight.

Second, compassion depends on the way in which any plight is understandable because of shared humanity. We may experience compassion because we see in the other person that which could foreseeably affect ourselves. It is not that we have to have experienced the same predicament; nor are we focused on our own needs. It is, rather, that we can see the way in which this plight resonates with our sense of what it is to face such a difficulty in life. There is a connection here between compassion and empathy.

Third, compassion is different from pity or sympathy. Pity and sympathy suggest that we may feel for the other, but because we recognize that we are not in such a situation and, whether through good fortune or our own efforts, think we are unlikely to be. So there is an element of condescension or patronization in these responses. In contrast, compassion reflects a grasp of the way in which this could happen to oneself. This is an important point, because those who emphasize *human dignity* or *human rights* may sometimes find the idea of compassion unhelpful. Measures to meet people's plights, such as policies or institutions, have arisen from a social and political response to such needs that then creates expectations of rights – we do not depend on having another person recognize our plight if a policy or service exists to help people with this problem, we show that we fit the criteria. However, if compassion is understood in the rounded sense of a common recognition of human need, then this can provide a powerful force to encourage the development of appropriate policies and institutions to meet such needs. It can even supply the moral basis for the people professions themselves.

Fourth, what may be regarded as a plight can differ between contexts. For example, the suffering of a child may be great over a matter that we might expect an adult to accept as a minor misfortune. Another example can be found in the way that our interests and personal concerns may make a loss of something minor to one person but a tragedy to another. This may also have a cultural component, as what is significant for a person from one culture may not be recognized by a person from another as having any value. For these reasons, both the scale and the meaning of a plight vary according to who is experiencing it.

Fifth, Nussbaum (2001, pp. 311–312) argues that compassion distinguishes those people who bear no fault for their plight from those who do; or, if there is a reason to attach blame, the plight is out of proportion to it. This is, perhaps, the most contentious part of her approach to this concept. While we may agree that some tragic predicaments are unjust (this may even make them appear more tragic), a wide variety of views will be found as to where the line may be drawn between those that are unjust and those that are not. There are those who will agree that when people create their own misfortune, through taking risks that can be foreseen or by failing to take reasonable care of their own actions, then a predicament is a just consequence. Others, however, may see the same situation as calling for compassion, because even making such poor judgements is part of the common human condition.

There are many situations in which different members of the people professions can see compassion differently. For example, a young patient in a hospital ward who has attempted suicide may evoke compassion in one nurse, while another regards the patient as wasting valuable health-care resources. Or, again, one teacher may see a student who continually hands assignments in late as having problems that call for compassion while another regards the student as lazy and uncooperative. Yet not all such distinctions arise from a lack of compassion. In a world of finite resources, a decision not to provide scarce expensive treatment to a person whose life-style choices have caused their ill-health and who appears unlikely to change their behaviour may be based on careful ethical deliberation. In this sort of situation, the limits of compassion come not from moral blame but from the principles of *consequential* ethics.

KEY TEXTS

- Halifax, J. (2012) 'A Heuristic Model of Enactive Compassion', *Current Opinion in Supportive and Palliative Care*, 6 (2): pp. 228–235

- Nussbaum, M. (2001) *Upheavals of Thought: The Intelligence of Emotions* (New York: Cambridge University Press), Part II
- Straughair, C. (2012) 'Exploring Compassion: Implications for Contemporary Nursing. Part 1', *British Journal of Nursing*, 21 (3): pp. 160–164

competence

SEE ALSO **beneficence; care; honesty; integrity; non-maleficence; respect; truth**

While at a surface level it might appear obvious that members of the people professions ought to be competent to undertake the roles they have, the idea that this should be an ethical issue is perhaps more complex. Yet there are three clear ways in which competence is a part of the ethical terrain of these professions.

First, the very idea of a profession says to other people in the community 'we can help you.' If, in fact, this is not the case because professionals lack the necessary skills and knowledge, then they fail the tests of *honesty, integrity* and *truth*; consequently, they also fail to *respect* the service user as a human person. That is, for a person to make a claim that he or she is able to help someone else when they should be aware that they do not have the necessary skills and knowledge is effectively to tell a lie. This is not a sound basis for a good professional relationship.

Second, engaging in a practice when someone does not have the required skills and knowledge may put the service user at risk of harm. Even if such harm is slight, to do this embodies neither *beneficence* or *non-maleficence*. In other words, not only does it not have an appropriate basis for seeking to do good but it also fails to take reasonable steps to avoid doing harm. It fails to exercise *duty of care*.

Third, the *ethics of care* approach identifies competence as part of a good caring relationship. This implies that the person who practices when not competent is being careless. Such a view goes beyond the everyday implications of lack of attention, as within this approach lack of care is construed as bad or wrong because it fails to engage in an ethical relationship.

The question of competence partly relates to education and training. Entry to professions tends to be based on defined minimum levels of skill and knowledge that have been tested. However, continuing professional education is also necessary for practitioners to maintain and further develop their competence. New knowledge and new procedures are constantly being developed, as well as practitioners moving into new areas of work. For all of these reasons, competence cannot be considered a matter of a once-and-for-all basic qualification but of constantly engaging with professional education as an ethical as well as a technical issue.

KEY TEXTS

- Bradshaw, A. (1996) 'Yes! There is an Ethics of Care: An Answer for Peter Allmark', *Journal of Medical Ethics*, 22 (1): pp. 8–12
- Kirsch, N.R. (20) 'Unsatisfying Satisfaction', *PT in Motion*, 2 (8): pp. 44–46
- Paganini, M.C. and Yoshikawa Ergy, E. (2011) 'The Ethical Component of Professional Competence in Nursing', *Nursing Ethics*, 18 (4): pp. 571–582

confidentiality

SEE ALSO autonomy; consequentialism; deontology; human rights; respect; trust

Modern professions regard the development of *trust* between practitioners and service users as vitally important. One of the ways in which this is achieved is through confidentiality. In order to perform their professional roles, practitioners need service users to provide information about themselves that they may wish not to disclose to others under normal circumstances. So this requires that professionals undertake not to share such information outside the helping relationship – these things are known only for the purpose of providing help and so are subject to 'special' expectations that would not attach to 'ordinary' relationships, such as with family or friends. In return for being provided with this intimate information, members of the people professions undertake not to share this knowledge to anyone that the service user does not want to have it. This is a *consequential* argument, as it is based on the goal of practitioners receiving full information that will enable them to respond to the best of their abilities.

There is also another argument for confidentiality, that of *respect* for the person. This is a type of *deontological* ethics, in which the practitioner has a moral duty to the person in her or himself, for no other reason than she or he is an *autonomous* human being. Disclosure of knowledge about the person without their consent, then, can be regarded as a violation of that person's dignity and capacity to make their own moral choices. When this is combined with the consequential argument in pluralist ethics, the principle of confidentiality is often seen to be very powerful. A classic statement of the principle of confidentiality, which has influenced social work, youth work and various forms of therapeutic practice, comes from Biestek (1959). However, it is important to recognize that Biestek proposes confidentiality as a principle of effective practice, so clearly including a consequential dimension, and clearly did not intend this to be absolute ethically.

Indeed, there are some important limits to this principle. In many legal systems, there is no absolute right for a service user to expect that information will not be provided to third parties (Bowles *et al.*, 2006). For instance, in some countries, there are expectations that certain sorts of criminal offences will be reported to the relevant authorities. The most notable example of this is in relation to the abuse of children. Beyond this, in other circumstances, courts may direct a professional practitioner to provide information. In such systems, a common response is to insist that information will only be shared with others either if the service user gives explicit agreement or if an order is actually made by court requiring disclosure. However, it is also important to recognize that in complex organizations information may routinely be shared among a team. Under such circumstances, service users should be aware of this and it is common to see this as a responsibility of all members of the team.

It is also the case that professional ethics may conflict with strongly held cultural expectations about the sharing of information. There are many parts of the world where such knowledge is regarded as belonging to families or *communities*, so under these conditions the practice of not disclosing can be experienced as culturally confronting. It may be, for example, that an elder, a parent or an older sibling is expected to make decisions about someone who is ill or experiencing other types of problems. However, this is not only a matter of 'the West versus the rest', but it can also be hotly debated in Western contexts. For example, confidentiality in work with adolescents can be a cause of dispute with parents who regard this as an infringement of their *responsibilities* and *human rights*. Therefore, how confidentiality is applied in practice requires careful thought and skill, balancing legal and policy requirements with cultural awareness and sensitivity.

KEY TEXTS
- Beauchamp, T.L. and Childress, J.F. (2009) *Principles of Biomedical Ethics*, 6th edn (New York: Oxford University Press), Chapter 8
- Collingridge, M. *et al.* (2001) 'Privacy and Confidentiality in Social Work', *Australian Social Work*, 54 (2): pp. 3–13
- Gournay, K. (1998) 'Ethical Issues in Mental Health Nursing' in W. Tadd (ed), *Ethical Issues in Nursing and Midwifery Practice* (Basingstoke: Macmillan)

confucian ethics (includes filial piety)

SEE ALSO community; duty; harmony; respect; responsibility; virtue

One of the major non-Western ethical traditions that impacts on the practice of people professions in many parts of the world is that of Confucianism. While it is not the only such tradition in Asia, it has a very large influence and shares many aspects with religious traditions such as Mahayana Buddhism, Shinto and Taoism. Of particular significance here is that Confucianism is a *community*-centred morality, which is often compared against the individualistic nature of Western ethics (Shun and Wong, 2004; Lai, 2006).

Of central importance in understanding Confucian ethics is the notion that we should ground an understanding of morality so as to maintain harmonious social relationships. This means that the primary concern is with *duties* and *responsibilities*. The model of such morality is the relationship of a son and a father, in which duty and responsibility of the son towards the father is grounded in respect for the authority of the senior person, but at the same time is necessarily associated also with upholding the father's duties and responsibilities to the wider community. Thus the individual self is understood to be interdependent and contextualized (Lai, 2006). This notion is usually translated into English as 'filial piety'. The gender-specific language reflects the original ideas and is common also in the Western philosophical traditions (such as the ancient Greeks) and many religious teachings. Also shared between Confucian ethics and the older Western traditions is the sense that the basis for morality is not the interests or rights of an individual but the overall well-being of the community. In addition, it is possible to draw parallels between Confucian ethics and the *virtue* approach that has its origins in Plato and Aristotle. For example, just as the ancient Greeks saw the interests of individuals and the community as convergent, so did Confucius and Mencius. The just person both promotes and is sustained by the just society in both traditions.

One of the ways in which this notion of filial piety can be seen to affect professional relationships is that the service user owes the practitioner a duty of respect. In turn, the practitioner has a responsibility to the service user to use their knowledge, skill and authority for the benefit of the service user and her or his family. Thus far, it would appear that there is little difference from other expectations: this is as it might be in Western, *African* or *Indigenous* contexts. The main difference, especially from Western ideas, is that the notion of *human rights* has no significance in filial piety at least as rights may be understood as properties of individuals, whether these are service users or professionals. In this sense, *autonomy* is understood as the capacity to reflect on choices of action within a context where if the exercise of choice is to be done well, it should be directed towards promoting harmonious social relationships. Thus Confucianism avoids the strong individualistic sense that is often regarded as characteristic of Western ethics.

For example, the practices that value being non-directive towards service users, such as various forms of counselling and psychotherapy, may be regarded from a Confucian perspective as inappropriate because practitioners are seen as failing in their responsibilities to give authoritative help. Thus it can be alleged that more concrete practices are more relevant and appropriate. This can apply in teaching, where the teacher who 'instructs' rather than 'guides self-directed learning' may be preferred, as well as in health and welfare fields where clinicians are likewise expected to 'give instruction' to their patients/clients.

Recent debates have characterized an East–West distinction in the provision of professional care services in terms of the dichotomy between Confucian and Western ethics. A particular example of this is in the field of care for older people, where Western policies and practices may be considered as inappropriate for Asian societies (Liu and Kendig, 2000). The assumption behind this debate is that 'Asian families care for their older members and Western families do not.' Whether this is an accurate portrayal of Western values depends on one's view of cultural history, as alternatives to family care are a relatively recent phenomenon, largely developing in their modern form in the late twentieth century (CE). However, that this has remained a point of debate from an Asian perspective reflects the perceived difference between Confucian and Western values as applied to an area of professional care. The recent development of institutional forms of care, such as nursing homes, in countries such as China and Japan suggest that these policies and practices reflect the impact of industrial society rather than an underlying difference of values. Thus, for the practitioner in this field, awareness of the specific understanding of culture by service users from whichever background presents a more appropriate starting point than gross generalizations.

KEY TEXTS

- Dean, E. (2001) 'Neo-Confucianism and Physiotherapy: The Mind-Body Spirit Connection', *Hong Kong Physiotherapy Journal*, 19; pp. 3–8
- Koh, E. and Koh, C. (2008) 'Caring for Older Adults: The Parables in Confucian Texts', *Nursing Science Quarterly*, 21 (4): pp. 365–368
- Tsai, D.F. (2005) 'The Bioethical Principles and Confucius' Moral Philosophy', *Journal of Medical Ethics*, 31 (3): pp. 159–163
- Yip, K. (2005) 'Chinese Concepts of Mental Health: Cultural Implications for Social Work Practice', *International Social Work*, 48 (4): pp. 391–407

consent (includes informed consent)

SEE ALSO **autonomy; deontology; duty; human agency; responsibility**

An important way in which a person can exercise their moral *autonomy* is through giving, or withholding, their consent to a particular intervention by a professional practitioner. Consent is the agreement of a person to participate in what is required in order to receive help, for the practitioner to perform the tasks necessary for help to be provided and so on.

In order for consent to be seen as an expression of moral autonomy, it must be given freely. That is, there should be no duress or coercion in the service users agreeing to receive help. For this to happen, it is widely agreed that the service must be informed as fully as possible about all aspects of what will happen. This includes the way in which the practitioner has assessed the problem or issue, the possible courses of action that can be taken and the reasons for choosing one rather than others (where there is more than one option), expected outcomes and possible risks and side-effects and their likelihood. Who is *responsible* for doing what should also be understood by service users, including whether they are expected to undertake particular actions. This is called 'informed consent' and is encountered in different ways in various professional contexts.

There are two arguments for limitations to the idea of consent. The first of these is that it is possible to give too much information to service users in circumstances where they cannot be expected to have sufficient background knowledge to make sense of it all. This view, which is a form of paternalism, is based on the idea that it is the *duty* of the professional practitioner to protect the service users from potential harm of being overloaded with information and so find it impossible to make choices in their own best interests. Against this, it can be argued that it is the responsibility of practitioners to develop ways of explaining their assessments, options for action, risks and so on in a language that a non-specialist can understand.

The second possible limitation to consent is that some tasks performed by members of the people professions are mandated by law. Service users are required to receive such services; they are not optional. Within this limitation, however, the principle of informed consent may operate in other ways. It remains morally as well as technically better for service users to understand what is to happen, what is expected of them and what can they expect of those who are working with them. The fact of receiving mandated interventions, for example, in the mental health or criminal justice systems, as well as in some respects school education, does not remove the *human agency* of the person and hence does not over-ride their autonomy. So even in these circumstances, it can be seen to be appropriate for both *deontological* and *consequential* reasons to use the principle of consent to the greatest extent possible.

KEY TEXTS
- Kaplan, L.E. (2009) 'A Conceptual Framework for Considering Informed Consent', *Journal of Social Work Ethics and Values*, 6 (3) (available at http://www.socialworker.com/jswve/content / view/130/69/)
- Saldov, M. and Kakai, H. (2004) 'The Ethics of Medical Decision Making with Japanese-American Elders in Hawai'i: Signing Informed Consent Forms without Understanding Them', *Journal of Human Behavior in the Social Environment*, 10 (1): pp. 113–130
- Tschudin, V. (2003) *Ethics in Nursing: The Caring Relationship*. 3rd edn (Oxford: Butterworth-Heinemann), Chapter 9

consequentialism

SEE ALSO justice; utilitarianism

A consequential approach to ethics is the one that considers what is good or right in terms of the outcomes of actions. If a given outcome is considered as good in some way, then the act that produces it will also be considered good. Conversely, if an act produces a bad outcome, then the act also is bad. This is one of the major elements of Western ethics and has had a major impact on professional ethics.

The most widely known example of consequential ethics is *utilitarianism*, which is considered in depth in a separate section. Indeed, there is sometime confusion between the two terms as they can be used synonymously. Utilitarianism is a type of consequential ethics, which evaluates what is good and right according to the balance of benefit or harm for everyone affected by an action (see discussion below). Other forms of consequential ethical judgements require different notions of the good to be applied. For example, ethical *egoism*, based on the pursuit of self-interest, views the pursuit of each person's interests as an ethical obligation and judges consequences against each person's view of what is good. In contrast, theories of *justice* provide a social view of determining the good in relation to the balance of outcomes for everyone who is affected (Freeman, 2000).

As social groups, professions do not usually favour ethical egoism and tend to emphasize a combination of utilitarian and justice principles. For example, questions about the way in which scare resources are allocated may be resolved using these ideas. If a practitioner only has five hours available, it takes one hour to see each service user and there are six people who need attention, then who is to be given time and who will not be seen? A consequential approach helps in thinking about this in terms of the expected outcomes for the service users, the outcome for the practitioner and the balance between the two. (This point is developed in more detail in the sections on justice and utilitarianism.)

KEY TEXTS

- Clifford, D. and Burke, B. (2009) *Anti-Oppressive Ethics and Values in Social Work* (Basingstoke: Palgrave Macmillan), Chapter 4
- Freeman, S.J. (2000) *Ethics: An Introduction to Philosophy and Practice* (Belmont CA: Wadsworth), Chapter 5
- Hinman, L.M. (2012) *Ethics: A Pluralistic Approach to Moral Theory* (Boston MA: Wadsworth), Chapter 5

courage

SEE ALSO **Confucian ethics; Indigenous ethics; principles; virtue**

Courage is a *virtue* that is widely recognized, not only in the Western ethical traditions but also in other systems, including *Confucian*
and other Asian, *African* and *Indigenous* perspectives. It refers to the capacity of a person to respond well to situations of risk, danger or threat. This is an ethical concept because it concerns the way in which people make judgements that for someone to display this characteristic is good. For example, the person who is able to overcome the fear of what will happen as a result of challenging someone in authority when the latter is making a mistake or is about to act badly may be considered courageous. Hinman (2012), a moral philosopher, argues that there are certain elements to this virtue: a right understanding of risks or threats; proper confidence in one's capacity to act and judgement about the action that follows. Thus, for example, the lack of courage may be thought of as cowardice (a deficiency of courage), while not stopping to make a considered judgement about the balance of risk and the likelihood of succeeding on one's actions is foolhardiness (an excess of courage). Hinman (2012, p. 262) gives the example of a person rushing into a burning building to save a baby who is trapped inside. Whether

this is courageous or foolhardy might depend on a perception of whether the baby can be rescued set against the life of the would-be rescuer. In comparison, to rush into a burning building to save an easily replaced inanimate object is much more likely to be considered foolhardy whatever the likelihood of success.

In professional contexts, courage is more likely to take the form of making judgements about pursuing what is right and opposing what is wrong when a tangible harm might happen to the person acting. Challenging one's superior because she or he is seen to be making a mistake is one such example, as in some circumstances this might have a detrimental effect on one's career. But speaking out against the opinion of a group of one's peers may also be a situation in which courage is needed. Comfortable working relationships and the maintenance of friendship are also values that can reasonably be held and these can be disrupted by courageously speaking out against something that is seen to be wrong. It may be courageous for a practitioner to choose an area of professional practice that is not popular or well regarded by their peers, especially if this is not well remunerated. Or choosing to work in parts of the world that are affected by conflict or natural disasters may require a different form of courage, even though this might be well regarded by one's peers: working under conditions of threat to one's personal safety would in this sense be an act of courage.

KEY TEXTS

- Crewe, S.E. (2004) 'A Time to Be Silent and a Time to Speak Up', *Reflections: Narratives of Professional Helping*, 10 (1): pp. 16–25
- Lindh, I. *et al.* (2010) 'Courage and Nursing Practice a Theoretical Analysis', *Nursing Ethics*, 17 (5): pp. 551–565
- Spence, D. and Smythe, L. (2007) 'Courage as Integral to Advancing Nursing Practice', *Nursing Praxis in New Zealand*, 23 (2): pp. 43–55
- Thomas, B. (2008) 'Seeing and Being Seen: Courage and the Therapist in Cross-Racial Treatment', *Psychoanalytic Social Work*, 15 (1): pp. 60–68

d

deontology (ethics of duty)

SEE ALSO **autonomy; codes of ethics; human agency; liberalism; principles; respect**

One of the central pillars of modern Western ethics, deontology concerns the ethics of *duty*. The term deontology is derived from the Greek word 'δεον', meaning 'duty' or 'that which is necessary'. However, when using the notion of duty it is vitally important to be clear about the object or objective to which duty is owed.

The most significant moral philosopher of deontology is Immanuel Kant (1724–1804 CE), whose ideas continue to have a major influence on professional ethics. Kant's ethics was developed over a lifetime of study and was interwoven with his philosophies of knowledge and of aesthetics. However, the main elements are summarized as shown in Table 2.

1.	The distinctive characteristic of humanity is the capacity for rationality.
2.	From this, it can be deduced that people have the capacity to think about what is right and wrong, or good and bad.
3.	Therefore to be treated as human means that every person should be regarded as a moral being.
4.	From this, every person owes every other person an absolute duty of respect.

TABLE 2 *Key characteristics of Kant's deontological ethics*

To set this out in the form of a rigorous principle, Kant proposed the 'categorical imperative'. This statement is categorical because it does not depend on any external variable factor (it is not an 'if' statement) and imperative because it is an instruction for an action. This is the famous claim that moral principles should be *universal* (see Table 3).

> 'Act only on that maxim through which you can at the same time will that it should become a universal law.'

TABLE 3 *The categorical imperative*
Kant, 1991 [1785], p. 84.

In other words, for an action to be good or right, it must be grounded in a principle that can be applied equally to everyone. A simple example is that it is not ethically acceptable to argue that I may tell a lie unless I allow that everyone else may also tell lies. However, to do so would undermine social relationships because it would destroy the integrity of human communication. Thus it is irrational and so morally self-defeating. Kant called this the test of universalism: that is, can the basis of an action be applied universally to everyone?

Kant then proceeded to think about how this imperative affects practical action. It is not sufficient, he stated, simply to claim that an act is good because I have chosen it (willed it); it must also be based on rationality rather than inclination. I should choose to act in a particular way because it is right, and not that I like the act for other reasons.

Following from this combination of rationality and universality, Kant concluded that all human beings are moral because they are rational, so no person can be seen simply as an object of someone else's subjective preferences. Thus, in the same way I want to be treated as a person who has ideas, interests, and can make moral choices, so I should also treat everyone else the same way. We are all, equally, moral subjects, for no other reason than that we are all capable of rationality. This then leads Kant to a second imperative, which he calls the 'practical imperative' (although it is categorical in the same sense as the previous imperative statement: it does not depend on an 'if' statement) (see Table 4).

In some ways this can be seen as a non-religious development from an idea that can be found in different forms in many of the

> 'Act in such a way that you always treat humanity, whether in your own person or in the person of any other, never simply as a means, but always at the same time as an end.'

TABLE 4 *The practical imperative*
Kant, 1991 [1785], p. 91.

world's major *religions,* such as 'do to others as you would have them do to you'.

This statement is the foundation of applied ethical principles such as *consent, human agency, human rights* and *respect.* If the idea of each person as a moral end in her or himself is taken seriously then it is not ethically permissible to do anything to them or for them, even if it is considered to be for their own good, unless that person agrees. Of course, in everyday life we may act in ways that affect others because we can make reasonable assumptions about their preferences. Yet the point is that under these conditions we have built up knowledge of the person – and if we find we are mistaken then it is very likely that we would apologize and make amends in some appropriate way, thus restoring their moral agency.

It is important to understand that the basis for Kantian ethics is rationality. Thus the duty in deontology is to ethical principles that are constructed from rational consideration. It is most emphatically *not* duty to the social authority of one's senior colleagues, managers or other people who may exert power over one's professional life. The defence of 'obeying orders' is morally incoherent from a Kantian perspective. Indeed, in this framework, one's ethical duty is to challenge those who give instructions that would require another person to be treated as a means to an end or where the principle behind the action could not be applied equally to others.

Historically, the breach of these duties has been seen in the involvement of professionals such as medical doctors, nurses, psychologists, social workers and teachers in the atrocities of the European Holocaust of the mid-twentieth century (CE) (e.g. see Johnstone, 1994, pp. 19–23). For most members of these and other professions the realities in everyday practice are less extreme. Yet from a deontological perspective this does not absolve any practitioner from the difficult *responsibility* of ensuring that in all that is done other people are treated as moral ends in themselves and that principles behind actions can be extended to everyone. Breaches of these imperatives can be seen in failures to give full information in obtaining consent, in not providing service users with information about all available options, in not asking service users about their view of what is happening to or for them or in general failing to treat people with dignity and respect.

Similarly, the notion of duty to one's family and friends is not a part of the deontological approach. While such a moral position may be seen positively in terms of the virtue of *loyalty*, or as an expression of *filial piety*, the particularity of such values through being part of specific relationships makes it impossible to use them as universal principles in a deontological manner. Performing an act out of duty to friends or family is regarded, within this approach, as 'nepotism', with very strong negative implications. For the deontologist attachment to such values does not take away the moral *responsibility* that each person has for her or his own actions.

Deontological ethics is very demanding. Acting on this basis can sometimes require *courage, honesty*, persistence and determination. It also necessitates clear thinking about the rationality of moral responses and ideas in practical situations. For example, if our role involves encouraging someone to make a decision, where the person is fearful and uncertain because of what is happening in their lives, but we need to do so quickly and not all options seem equally good to us, how do we act to treat someone as a moral agent? Or, how do I accomplish some very important research work that has the potential to help, even save the lives of, many other people if my potential subjects exercise their capacity to refuse to participate? Again, is it realistic to question my senior colleague who has directed me to do something that I believe to be against the service users' wishes, because that colleague can affect my career when they make a recommendation about me in the future?

If deontological ethics is to form the foundation for the professions, it means that practitioners should integrate this into all aspects of their work, so that the way in which decisions are made and implemented is routinely based on the categorical and practical imperatives. Kant argued that there should be no exceptions to a moral duty. This is not necessarily followed by contemporary Kantians, as the everyday world requires that we make judgements (Hinman, 2012). A clear example provided by Hinman (2012, p. 166) is that in many countries where road traffic laws are enforced it is permitted for an ambulance to go above a speed limit or to proceed through a stop-sign, when taking a critically ill person to an emergency facility. However, such exceptions do not undermine the general deontological approach if they are always exceptional (i.e. not really part of everyday routines) and that by making an exception the moral standing of people and the maxims that inform action (such as 'when driving it is necessary always to conform to road traffic laws') are promoted more broadly.

KEY TEXTS

- Banks, S. (2012) *Ethics and Values in Social Work*. 4th edn (Basingstoke: Palgrave Macmillan), Chapter 2
- Beauchamp, T.L. and Childress, J.F. (2009) *Principles of Biomedical Ethics*. 6th edn (New York: Oxford University Press), Chapter 9
- Freeman, S.J. (2000) *Ethics: An Introduction to Philosophy and Practice* (Belmont, CA: Wadsworth), Chapter 6
- Rachels, J. (2010) *The Elements of Moral Philosophy*. 6th edn (New York: McGraw-Hill), Chapters 9 and 10

dignity

SEE ALSO **deontology; honour; respect**

When a person is treated with great *respect* and in a way that demonstrates that she or he is regarded as having high moral standing then we may say that the person is being treated with dignity. This implies that the person receives the esteem of others and her or his humanity is recognized. In terms of Kantian *deontology*, dignity is a quality that describes the absolute inherent worth of each person as a moral being. Dignity is also the opposite of ridicule or humiliation. As an aspect of a person's character, it suggests that the person conducts her or himself in a way that is congruent with receiving respect and esteem. So from this ethical standpoint, if a person lacks dignity it should be because the person her or himself has chosen to act otherwise and not because dignity has been taken away by the acts of others.

This notion has been criticized as being 'useless' because it lacks precision and so has no place in the everyday world of practice (Macklin, 2003). One example cited is the idea of 'death with dignity', which Macklin asserts has no meaning. Against this view the idea is defended by Schroeder (2010), who points to four elements that are combined in everyday usage, mixing notions of inherent worth, status, well-mannered behaviour and meritorious character. Thus dignity is a way of connecting ideas that have their roots in different principles rather than a principle in itself. Killmister (2010) argues that in contemporary professional practice, occasions on which the concept of dignity is opaque can be disentangled by integrating the Kantian meaning of inherent worth with a combination of behaviour and character that she sees as 'aspirational' (what people would like to be in terms of who they are and what they do).

A concrete example of dignity in practice is described by Browne (1995), a white Canadian nurse, from her work with Inuit people, especially women. Browne describes how she discovered some important cross-cultural values around the idea of respect, in which providing women with dignity in the way that physical examinations were conducted enhanced working with people from a different cultural background. This included privacy as well as taking time to clear about why certain procedures were necessary to conduct examinations.

KEY TEXTS

- Browne, A.J. (1995) 'The Meaning of Respect: A First Nations' Perspective', *Canadian Journal of Nursing Research*, 27 (4): pp. 95–110
- Killmister, S. (2010) 'Dignity, Not Such a Useless Concept', *Journal of Medical Ethics*, 36 (3): pp. 160–164
- Macklin, R. (2003) 'Dignity Is a Useless Concept', *British Medical Journal*, 327 (7429): pp. 1419–1420
- Schroeder, D. (2010) 'Dignity: One, Two, Three, Four, Five, Still Counting', *Cambridge Quarterly of Healthcare Ethics*, 19 (1): pp: 118–125

discourse ethics

SEE ALSO codes of ethics; responsibility; truth

This concept is based on the social and political philosophy of Habermas (1990). It is grounded in the notion of democracy. For Habermas a democratic society must be one in which people have the opportunity to engage freely in dialogue about what is good and right. Habermas seeks to build ethics on practical discourse, which is the way that people talk about things. Ethical discourse is concerned with *truth*, but there are different facets of truth that must be taken into account. Habermas distinguishes between truth as what is factually true, what is normatively right and what is subjectively truthful. From this understanding he proposes a principle of discourse ethics, in which 'only those norms can claim to be valid that meet (or could meet) with the approval of all affected in their capacity as participants in a practical discourse' (Habermas, 1990, p. 93).

One way in which the notion of discourse ethics can be explained by reference to the professions is in the issue of research using human subjects and the ethic of *informed consent*. For example, while it may be factually correct that there is only a very slight risk to subjects through participating in a particular project this does not outweigh the norm of informed consent. For the research team, or indeed the wider professional community, to decide that side-stepping consent in such an instance is acceptable simply because it helps the research to proceed will not do in terms of discourse ethics. To act in this way would be a misuse of professional knowledge to distort the practical discourse – in other words, it skews the ethical dialogue in favour of those who have both the technical knowledge and the vested interest in a particular outcome (in this instance, the collection of research data). Thus, in these terms, it would be both subjectively untruthful and also undemocratic. In addition, because of the latter aspect, it could also be seen as undermining the notion of *justice*. For this reason, even though the researchers may accurately grasp the objective truth of the degree of possible physical harm, in ethical terms their actions could only be understood as deceptive, coercive and unjust. Habermas' concept can also be seen as drawing on Kantian *deontology* because unjust and undemocratic action also leads to some people (professionals and researchers) treating others (such as service users) simply as a mean to achieve research goals in which the service users may have had no say. This argument applies across all practices because, by definition, they affect people who are not members of the particular professions.

A more complex example is encountered in situations where service users are compelled to receive the interventions of a practitioner, such as those mandated by law. However, while in one sense it may well be that some service users might not give voluntary approval to particular norms, the statutory nature of the intervention is likely in itself to be a reflection of the way in which the wider society asserts a particular set of norms against which disagreement may be possible but is not seen as acceptable. These are normative values concerning acts that are perceived as harmful to other people. Child abuse and domestic and family violence are clear examples of this. There are many situations in which practical discourse may include voices arguing that such matters are acceptable because they are 'normal' or 'natural'. However, in many societies in recent decades these acts have come to be regarded as unacceptable because they are harmful to people (in these cases children and, mostly, women) who are vulnerable. Here it is the public nature of the discourse around these issues that renders it democratic, given that agreement by all who are affected is impossible to achieve. Thus other principles, such as justice, come into play and inform the way in which the ethics of involuntary receipt of professional services is addressed.

Hugman (2005) argues that discourse ethics also provides the basis for thinking about formal professional ethical statements, such as codes of ethics. It suggests that to be internally consistent such collective statements of values and principles ought to be generated through processes of deliberation in which all those who are affected may have a voice. In practice this tends to be done by representative structures, such as ethics committees, but the implication is that ethics is not simply a matter of applying a technical document, but is better understood as a conversation in which all are participating. So, although many may choose to listen rather than to speak, this discursive view of ethics argues for the potential of any member of a profession to be involved in the ethical dialogue of that profession and, indeed, for the moral *responsibility* of all members to be aware of and engaged with the ethics of their profession.

KEY TEXTS
- Degner, L.F. (2002) 'Discourse, Ethics and Decision-Making: Lessons From the Cancer Wars', *Canadian Journal of Nursing Research*, 34 (3): pp. 9–13
- Houston, S. (2010) 'Discourse Ethics' in M. Gray and S.A. Webb (eds), *Ethics and Value Perspectives in Social Work* (Basingstoke: Palgrave Macmillan)
- Willette, C. (1998) 'Practical Discourse as Policy Making: An Application of Habermas' Discourse Ethics within a Community Mental Health Setting', *Canadian Journal of Community Mental Health*, 17 (2): pp. 27–38

e

emotion and moral sentiment

SEE ALSO care (ethics of); compassion; fairness; values

One of the effects of the emphasis on rationality in modern Western ethics has been the exclusion of considerations of emotion. While the emotions may be considered as facts about the human condition, such as when they form preferences that are then seen as a way of defining what is good in some types of *utilitarianism*, references to emotion or sentiment more generally are rejected as the basis for considering norms in both *deontological* and *consequential* approaches. The reason for this is that emotions and sentiments are subjective. In other words, they come from within each individual (a subject) and so have no way of being compared against a standard that is separate from the views of that person. An example of this is found in the idea that 'beauty is in the eye of the beholder'. (In contrast, both deontology and consequentialism can be regarded as objective and so claimed as free from bias, because they are based on values that are independent of a person.)

Yet other approaches to ethics have either recognized or even incorporated emotion as part of the way in which thinking about how what is good and right can be defined and understood, as well as in considering the way in which ethical deliberations can be made. The ancient Western and Eastern approaches to ethics recognized that emotions are an integral part of what it is to be human and that accounts of good and right must incorporate these. It may be that emotions require careful nurturing and to be held in balance by other factors such as reason, but not that they should be removed from consideration. For example, this can be seen in the ethics of both Confucius (551–479 BCE) and Socrates (469–399 BCE).

Not only are emotions considered by some approaches as problematic because they are regarded as irrational, but also emotions are often seen as introducing a problem of partiality to ethics. That is, emotions and sentiment can be regarded as the basis for many aspects of human life that provide difficulties when an ethical principle is applied across a society or social group (such as a profession). Family relationships, friendship and other close emotional connections may create obligations or give a particular tone to ethical deliberations that might lead to accusations of favouritism or nepotism. Formal ethics, such as in a profession, is seeking to emphasize impartiality so that principles such as *fairness* or *justice* can operate. This points to the fact that such ethical concepts concern the morality of public spaces and relationships precisely in order to remove the moral considerations that might come into play in 'private life'. Against this, it has been argued that if someone is expected to ask whether they should favour a person with whom they have a close relationship then this is requiring them to have 'one thought too many' (Williams, 1981, p. 18). This means that there are conditions in which it is simply good that one might favour one person over another on the basis of emotion and relationship. Williams' example is that of a man who chooses to save his wife from danger in circumstances where two people are threatened and only one can be saved. Of course, he states, anyone who did not save their spouse or close friend instead of another person has lost something of their own humanity. The problem here is that in professional life we are largely not dealing with such issues and questions of fairness, justice and other impartial notions tend to have priority. The medical practitioner or nurse who treated a family member before an unknown member of the public would be usually be seen to have acted badly when triage suggests the unknown person is in greater need, or in conditions of equal need had sought attention first. The same would be said for the school teacher or youth worker who favoured their own children.

At a different level, Nussbaum (2001) argues that emotions are part of our intelligence and cannot be ignored. Whether things make us happy or sad, delighted or disgusted, pleased or angry, proud or ashamed and so on, tell us about our own *values*. For this reason, we should attend to our emotions in order to understand and to think more deeply about our choices and actions. Nussbaum is particularly concerned with *compassion* as the intelligent emotion experienced in response to the suffering of others. This has clear implications for those professions that may be regarded as 'caring' or 'helping'. Indeed, it immediately raises the question of whether the notion of *care* can be applied accurately if compassion is lacking. For example, nurses in an emergency room dealing with people who are drunk, covered in vomit and uncooperative, or the social worker counselling a man who has sexually abused his child, have to have a well-developed ethical sense of their emotions if they are to undertake such tasks well. This is not to 'excuse' behaviour that is widely regarded as unacceptable, but concerns the necessity of developing and maintaining the capacity to respond to the humanity in a person who is likely to be generating disgust and anger in many others.

It is not that we should have to feel the same sort of emotions for someone who is a service user that we do for our family and friends, but that our orientation to caring practice has to be grounded in a sense of emotional engagement with the common humanity of those who are suffering. Moreover, when we find ourselves unwilling or unable to act to care for someone who is suffering, emotional intelligence requires ethical reflection on our judgements. It is more difficult to provide care for someone about whom we feel anger, disgust, envy or shame. For this reason the ethics of public and private spaces cannot be clearly separated if emotions are taken seriously.

KEY TEXTS

- Arnd-Caddigan, M. and Pozzuto, R. (2009) 'The Virtuous Social Worker: The Role of "Thirdness" in Ethical Decision Making', *Families in Society: The Journal of Contemporary Social Services*, 90 (3): pp. 323–328
- Burks, D.J. and Kobus, A.M. (2012) 'The Legacy of Altruism in Health Care: The Promotion of Empathy, Prosociality and Humanism', *Medical Education*, 46 (3): pp. 317–325
- Nussbaum, M. (2001) *Upheavals of Thought* (New York: Cambridge University Press), Part II

equality

SEE ALSO **fairness; justice; social justice**

Human beings differ from each other in many ways. Some of these differences are biological, such as sex or physical strength; some are psychological including intelligence and personality and some are social and cultural. At the same time many of the *principles* and *values* that underpin the ethics of the professions emphasize the way in which all human beings have equal moral worth. Both *deontology* and *utilitarianism* lead to this conclusion and support it in different ways. More recent emphasis on *human rights* and *social justice* strengthen the value of equality seen in this way.

Although the broad notion of equality is shared between approaches there are different ways in which it is understood. Banks (2012, p. 50) distinguishes between three types of equality: treatment; opportunity; result (outcome). The first of these, equality of treatment, requires that practitioners respond to each service user (whether this is an individual, a family, a group or a community) in the same way as any other service user. Of course, each set of needs can be expected to be different, but in terms of the attention given, treating people with *respect* and prioritizing between service users on the basis of type of need each service user with their distinct needs can be treated equally.

Equality of opportunity is the aspect that is perhaps best recognized in public debate in Western countries. This understanding of equality regards disadvantage experienced by some people to be caused by social arrangements, so that equality can be achieved by changing these arrangements. This may include ensuring that criteria for providing services do not contain elements that are easier for some social groups to achieve and which do not relate directly to the provision of the service. In the employment of practitioners the same principle can be applied, such as by ensuring that factors used to select are not biased towards certain types of people in ways that are irrelevant to a position. Further than this, some remedial measures may be taken to mitigate social structural disadvantage, a process that is known as affirmative action or positive discrimination.

Equality of result or outcome is when two people or groups can achieve the same valued ends although their circumstances may differ. The example given by Banks (2012, p. 63) is that of two people who need nursing home care, where the same high-quality care is made available even though one is very wealthy and the other in poverty. This is achieved in some countries through tax-funded support for such services, either means tested as the basis for allocating public funds or universally available in order to avoid stigma.

In countries where government policies seek to reduce or eliminate inequality through an emphasis on equality in terms of treatment and opportunity, some critics argue that this potentially places an undue constraint on individual *freedom* (e.g. in being required to pay tax to support someone else living well in a nursing home). However, one of the most influential modern theories of *justice*, that of John Rawls (1921–2002 CE), seeks to balance the competing demands of freedom and equality by spelling out two basic principles. Rawls (1972) wishes to preserve the greatest possible freedom for each person consistent with the same amount of freedom for all others, while at the same time allowing inequality only insofar as it benefits everyone and exists under conditions that are open to everyone to the same extent. Equality of treatment and equality of opportunity are now widely regarded as norms in many professional contexts. Equality of result or outcome remains more contentious, largely because for many people it is seen as achievable only by placing undue constraint on freedom.

This understanding of equality, which has been highly influential, sees it not in terms of people 'getting the same' but of a complex *fairness* (Gray, 1996). From this point of view, it may be entirely reasonable that someone else gets more help than I do because they have different needs. In practice, this is how many situations in education, health, social welfare and human services are decided. Rationing systems are very common, as triage in health services where levels of patient need is used to determine clinical priorities. In this way of thinking advantages such as being able to pay to be at the front of the queue are considered unfair and so are not used to determine service responses. However, at the same time various commentators continue to observe that even after allowing for factors such as the reluctance of members of certain social groups to seek professional assistance, awareness of services and unequal geographical distribution of services, services are not always fairly distributed. Women, members of ethnic minorities, people with disabilities and members of other minority groups frequently receive lower levels of services in Western countries (Beauchamp and Childress, 2009, pp. 250–253; Clifford and Burke, 2009, pp. 208–212).

KEY TEXTS

- Beauchamp, T.L. and Childress, J.F. (2009) *Principles of Biomedical Ethics* (New York: Oxford University Press), Chapter 7
- Kangasniemi, M. (2010) 'Equality as a Central Concept of Nursing Ethics', *Scandinavian Journal of Caring Sciences*, 24 (4): pp. 824–832
- Reisch, M. (2002) 'Defining Social Justice in a Socially Unjust World', *Families in Society: The Journal of Contemporary Social Services*, 83 (4): pp. 343–354

ethical egoism

SEE ALSO altruism; autonomy; courage; existential ethics; freedom; human agency

The arguments of ethical egoism sometimes claim that because people tend to act in their own interests it is good that people be *free* to do so. However, as Rachels (2010) and Hinman (2012) both argue, this claim requires further investigation, because it confuses a descriptive statement, 'what is' (people tend to act in a particular way), with a normative claim concerning 'what ought to be' (it is good that people act in this way). That people do tend to act in their own interests does not by itself make it good or right.

One possibility that would support the moral assertion of ethical egoism is that it promotes *autonomy* and *freedom*. This view was proposed by Nietzsche (1844–1900 CE) and Rand (1905–1982 CE), who saw a value such as *altruism* as a form of moral weakness because, they argued, it distorts the achievement of full human potential. From this perspective, a truly human life is the one in which a person can pursue those things that they value without having to sacrifice anything to suit others. In this approach altruism is seen as being valued by people who value themselves too little. Rachels (2010, pp. 71–73) summarizes Rand's view in these terms: altruism demands that a person sacrifice her or his life and that such a demand is, therefore, an argument against the moral value of persons. Ironically, at the same time, Rand appears to say that altruism is dishonest because it serves the interests of those who are weak. By expecting a virtuous person to give up something of her or himself for others who do not live well serves only the interests of those who would rather someone else exerted the effort to meet everyone's needs.

One aspect of ethical egoism would appear to have a possible contribution to make to professional ethics. If achieving self-interested autonomy is accepted as an ideal moral position, then the goal of empowerment might be regarded as a means to achieve this (e.g. compare with Adams, 2008). When empowered people can be expected to pursue their own interests and for the ethical egoist this is a moral as well as a practical gain. Yet the very act of providing assistance by itself is caught in the problem of self-interest. If ethical egoism is correct, then the professional is acting in such a way so as to make her or himself feel good and not because of compassion, empathy or any other directed value (see Rachels, 2010, p. 70).

However, while this description of empowerment may be sufficient for a purely technical or material service, for anything concerning the 'person' of the service user it is inadequate, as it says nothing about issues of *justice, fairness* and other moral questions that are raised by the nature of the professions themselves. These are moral qualities that apply to the society as a whole and not simply to an individual. To be consistent, the ethical egoist should not be concerned about society. So, at the very best, such a position if applied consistently would reduce the professional–service user relationship to one of a formal business contract, which is at odds with the values that underpin education, health, social service and so on (compare with Koehn, 1994). Professions in these areas are concerned with goals such as empowerment not only for the benefit of individual service users (although they are concerned with individuals), but also *at the same time* with the way in which their services contribute to a better society.

KEY TEXTS
- Hinman, L.M. (2012) *Ethics: A Pluralistic Approach to Moral Theory* (Boston MA: Wadsworth), Chapter 4
- Rachels, J. (2010) *The Elements of Moral Philosophy*. 6th edn (New York: McGraw-Hill), Chapter 5

evil

SEE ALSO **religion and ethics; virtue**

For many people, especially in Western contexts, this notion will probably be associated with *religion*. However, it is also used by moral philosophers working in other traditions and has something to contribute to discussions about the people professions. Hugaas (2010) defines the concept quite specifically in relation to acts as opposed to agents, in other words to what people do rather than who they are. Both *deontological* and *utilitarian* criteria can assist our thinking here, as both these approaches focus on actions. However, Hugaas actually goes further and argues that a *pluralist* reading of the two together is necessary as each contains distorting features if left on its own. Thus it is important to consider both volition (the act is chosen by an agent) and consequence (a serious moral harm must happen). Nor does it matter whether an act was intended to cause serious moral harm, 'only that it was *foreseeable*' (Hugaas, 2010, p. 268 – emphasis in original).

The third element in this understanding is that the harms addressed by the notion of evil are moral in nature. It does not refer to other types of injury, such as material loss, unless such harm also has a moral dimension to it. This aspect requires a volitional agent that is the source of the act – for example, a natural disaster is overwhelmingly harmful to people and other forms of life, but it cannot be considered evil because it lacks this characteristic. Alongside this element, the notion of evil must also be reserved for those acts that particularly cause serious moral harm. Hinman (2012) concurs with this point and uses the term 'egregious' (beyond normal boundaries, outside expected limits) to describe the sorts of harm that might be considered as evil.

Although producing their analyses separately, in their discussions of evil Hugaas and Hinman direct our attention to comparable sorts of acts. Interpersonal violence, child abuse, rape, torture and terrorism are examples of such acts (and may often be combined). They produce extreme moral harm as well as physical, emotional, psychological and spiritual trauma. Hinman (2012, p. 51) also makes the point that in many instances such acts are perpetrated against people who are relatively powerless, with women, children and ethnic or racial minorities overwhelmingly victims of such acts in all parts of the world. Practitioners encounter such events and their impact in clinics and hospitals, social work offices, schools and youth centres, often as the cause of some of the most demanding and difficult work that must be done.

In the nineteenth century (CE) in Western countries the notion of opposing 'social evils' was a strong motivating force in the professionalization of many of the occupations that might now be recognized as people professions. This use of the concept does not conform to the requirement that the notion of evil applies to volitional acts. However, the social conditions that were considered evil were those that generated serious social problems in human lives and so caused egregious moral harm. Child labour and child prostitution, human trafficking of other kinds, endemic crime, the widespread abuse of drugs and alcohol and other aspects of life in the early industrial cities were the product of poverty, social dislocation, insecure employment and other effects of the industrial revolution. The term social evil has also been used in other parts of the world in the late twentieth century to describe the same issues and problems, arising from the same causes. This can be seen as appropriate as these effects of social change are the product of human action, they are not 'natural disasters', and they can be addressed by policies and practices including those of the people professions. In this sense the concept of evil can inform the moral basis for such professions, especially when working in conditions of extreme human need.

KEY TEXTS
- Allen, J.G. (2007) 'Evil, Mindblindness and Trauma: Challenges to Hope', *Smith College Studies in Social Work*, 77 (1): pp. 9–31
- Erlingsson, C.L. (2011) 'Evil and Elder Abuse', *Nursing Philosophy*, 12 (4): pp. 248–261
- Hugaas, J.V. (2010) 'Evil's Place in the Ethics of Social Work', *Ethics & Social Welfare*, 4 (3): pp. 254–279
- Pellegrino, E.D. (2005) 'Some Things Ought Never to Be Done: Moral Absolutes in Clinical Ethics', *Theoretical Medicine and Bioethics*, 26 (6): pp. 469–486

existential ethics

SEE ALSO **courage; politics; religion and ethics; responsibility**

There have been very few attempts to apply existentialism in professional ethics. Indeed, this may be quite reasonable as the basis of existentialist philosophy is that each human being is morally *responsible* for her or his own life and must make what sense of it as they can. In such an understanding there are no fixed *duties* nor can what is good or right be considered simply from *consequences*. Existentialism derives originally from the work of the Danish philosopher Søren Kierkegaard (1813–1855 CE), for whom ethics is closely connected with *religious* thought, and was subsequently developed by Jean-Paul Sartre (1905–1980 CE) and his associates in France, for whom it could be said to have become a matter of *politics*.

The common thread of existentialist thought is that every person faces the moral choice of who she or he is and, from this, how she or he will act. The goal is to be as free as possible to live an 'authentic' life, in the sense of being true to oneself. Authenticity is the primary good and is opposed by 'bad faith', which can be understood as self-deception. To live in bad faith is to deny the capacity that people have for understanding their circumstances and taking action. So, saying 'there's nothing I can do' is not authentic if it does not recognize that this too is a choice. However, this does leave the impression that any choices are acceptable if the person lives with self-awareness and a sense of responsibility. This makes existentialism difficult to apply to many aspects of professional life where goals and choices are not necessarily free in this way.

Clifford and Burke (2009, pp. 149–155), writing in the field of social work, provide one rare example of a way in which existential ethics might be used in practice. They describe a practitioner who is faced with moral uncertainty in groupwork with young people, where a group member aged 13 acts offensively and then leaves the group in distress. The practitioner is aware of her responsibility not only to the young person but also to the other group members, so has to decide whether to leave the group to deal with the individual's distress or leave her to make her own way home – if, indeed, she goes home, which may become the ethical question that will be posed by others if it turns out that she does not. As it is described, the practitioner chooses to stay with the group, this action is 'authentic' in that it is not done in anger to punish the young person, nor does the practitioner act simply to protect herself from possible criticism. In that sense being authentic requires *courage* both in relation to oneself and to others, but this is done consciously and thoughtfully not casually.

KEY TEXTS

- Meiers, S.J. and Bauer, D.J. (2008) 'Existential Caring n the Family Health Experience', *Scandinavian Journal of Caring Sciences*, 22 (1): pp. 110–117
- Pascal, J. and Endacott, R. (2010) 'Ethical and Existential Challenges Associated with Cancer Diagnosis', *Journal of Medical Ethics*, 36 (5): pp. 279–283
- Ressler, A.B. (2006) 'An Existential Examination of Health Care Ethics', *International Journal for Human Caring*, 10 (1): pp. 61–67

f

fairness

SEE ALSO equality; justice; social justice; virtue

Fairness can be understood as the achievement of a balance between competing claims. It may also be applied both to people as a *virtue*, as in 'she's a fair supervisor', or to actions or events as a *principle*, as in 'that is a fair decision'. Therefore, in some sense, it is associated with *justice*, which also involves balance and has both virtue and principle dimensions. However, the problem with the idea of fairness is reflected in different ways in which it is explained. MacIntyre (1998) identifies fairness with distributive justice (as discussed elsewhere in this volume), that is with a balanced spread of goods (moral and material) across a community. In contrast, Hinman (2012) associates it with impartiality of the kind proposed within *deontology*.

With regard to fairness as a virtue, although that notion refers to people's character, it is actually demonstrated in the way in which people apply a balance in their judgements to decisions or choices that they have to make. For example, a fair teacher is the one who encourages in ways that recognize which students need to be encouraged, or who grades work in ways that are considered and understood by students, or who uses penalties in way that appear to students to be proportionate to wrong acts on their part. A fair manager or supervisor is the one who asks members of a team to perform tasks of which they are capable, who is seen as not asking too much of one person and too little of another and so on. These examples contain elements of both distributive justice and a sort of impartiality, even though the outcome may actually not be an exact equality. The student with a lower grade may see the teacher as fair because her or his judgement reflects the extent to which the student grasped the subject, or the team member with a larger caseload this month sees the supervisor as fair because she knows that she had a lower load earlier in the year.

As a description of decisions or actions, fairness can be understood in much the same way – this is, what a fair person does. It is possible to separate the two, insofar as a person who is considered fair might at times act in a way that is regarded as unfair by others, or the opposite may happen and an 'unfair person' is fair in a particular instance.

Possibly because of its apparent vagueness and the way in which it needs to be explained by reference to other concepts, there is little discussion about fairness in the professional ethics literature. Yet in most circumstances, it might be expected that service users are more likely to use an ordinary understanding of this notion than the more complex idea of justice in considering their interactions with practitioners or organizations. So it might repay the people professions to give more thought to this concept in the discussion of applied ethics.

KEY TEXTS

- Braveman, P.A. *et al.* (2011) 'Health Disparities and Health Equity: The Issue Is Justice', *American Journal of Public Health*, 101 (Supplement 1): pp. S149–S155
- Kirby, J. (2010) 'Enhancing the Fairness of Pandemic Critical Care Triage', *Journal of Medical Ethics*, 36 (12): pp. 758–761
- Sheppard, M. (2002) 'Mental Health and Social Justice: Gender, Race and Psychological Consequences of Unfairness', *British Journal of Social Work*, 32 (6): pp. 779–797

feminist ethics

SEE ALSO care (ethics of); emotion; justice; politics

Underlying feminist approaches to ethics is the analysis of society and interpersonal relationships from the perspective of gender. This analysis shows that in most societies social power and advantage is distributed unequally between the sexes, with men being generally advantaged (when all other factors are accounted for). The social systems and ideologies that sustain this as natural are called patriarchy, which literally means 'rule by the father' but is used to mean rule by men.

A central aspect of the feminist argument in ethics is that historically the dominant voices in moral philosophy have been those of men (Jaggar, 1992). It is not that women have been entirely absent from such debates, but that patriarchy operates to make theirs a minority, subjugated voice (Hoagland, 1996). From a feminist perspective, this can explain the exclusion of emotions and sentiments from ethics and the tendency for rationalism to dominate. Thus ethics, whether in Western, Asian or other traditions, has tended to be the morality of public life and in the modernist era to emphasize technical approaches to ethical issues. Thus notions of contract, rules and duties, rights and so on form the stock of ethical debates, while relationships, caring and other values that consider people's needs are either ignored or treated as subsidiary.

One of the major contributions to ethics in the twentieth century (CE) from feminist analysis has been the *ethics of care*. Initially proposed by Gilligan (1982), using the notion of 'voice' to describe the distinctive moral perspective of women has become a critical contribution to recent ethical thought. The focus on women's experience as the basis for ethics raises the question of whether all women necessarily share common values and, in corollary, whether men are not capable of engaging with the world in these terms. The view that women and men are necessarily different in this way is called 'essentialism', because it assumes an essential characteristic or nature in what it is to be female or male. Against this, the more dominant view has become more subtle, seeing women and men as differently positioned socially but both as capable of basing their ethics on relationships, experience, reflection and other elements that make it possible for men to 'be caring' and for women not to be so. This is significant, because the essentialist view creates a risk that women are then seen as locked into 'traditional roles', which perpetuate the very disadvantages that feminism seeks to expose and challenge (Held, 1993; Hoagland, 1996).

Not all feminist ethics is ethics of care. For example, in bioethics and social ethics a major contribution of feminist approaches has been to raise questions about the exclusion of women from ethical theory, debate and the implications of ethics in decision-making. The integration of the personal and *political* dimensions of moral thought is the central feature of feminist ethics. For example, the work of Kuhse (1997) approaches feminism from a *utilitarian* perspective, while Held (1993) and Tronto (1993) consider feminist issues from the values of *justice* and Nussbaum's (2000) work represents a *liberal* view of feminism. A different paradigm is offered from lesbian ethics (Hoagland, 1996), arguing that even feminist ethics is still engaging with the terms set by patriarchal cultures and structures. This leads to an argument for the development of an understanding of women's *agency* that is entirely separate from ethical traditions as currently conceived, largely achieved by separating women's lives from those of men.

Wise (1995) cautions that although the critique of social relations provided by feminist theory is accurate, application to practice in the people professions is far from straightforward, notably because of the *power* exercised by professionals. Using the example of practice with a woman who is subject to domestic violence and whose children are deemed to be at risk because of the way she has responded to her situation, Wise notes that practitioners who work from a feminist ethic may face the dilemma of challenging the world-views of women who do not see patriarchal social relations and structures as the source of their problems. As Wise puts it, 'I thought the men in her life were a problem; she wanted her violent husband back...' (1995, p. 110). Wise then asks whether practices that focus on 'empowerment' based on the word-view of the practitioner is simply treating women as suffering from 'false consciousness' and so needing to have her values altered. This would effectively be a self-contradiction as in seeking to assist women to develop non-oppressed agency would then seem to require that others (even if feminists) set the terms for how this should be achieved.

More widely, feminist perspectives also note that many of the people professions historically have been 'women's professions', most especially allied health, nursing, social work and teaching. Thus the ascription of the idea of 'semi-profession' to allied health, nursing, social work, school teaching and youth work was challenged as a subordination that derived from the historical tendency for these to be professions that are largely populated by women (Witz, 1992; Fry and Johnstone, 2002). While this challenge has only partly been successful, in some instances it has produced the possibility of different relationships between professional groups as well as between women and men within professions.

KEY TEXTS

- Curren, R. (ed) 'Symposium on Sentimentalist Moral Education', *Theory and Research in Education*, 8 (2): pp. 123–197
- Simpson, C. (2002) 'Hope and Feminist Care Ethics: What Is the Connection?' *Canadian Journal of Nursing Research*, 34 (2): pp. 81–94
- Stocker, S.S. (2005) 'The Ethics of Mutuality and Feminist Relational Therapy', *Women and Therapy*, 28 (2): pp. 1–15
- Wise, S. (1995) 'Feminist Ethics in Practice' in R. Hugman and D. Smith (eds), *Ethical Issues in Social Work* (London: Routledge)

fidelity

SEE ALSO honesty; loyalty; respect; trust; truth; virtue

Derived from the notion of faithfulness, fidelity is a *virtue* that has several dimensions. These include *loyalty, honesty* and *truth*. So, for example, when applied to non-moral goods, fidelity can be expressed in an appraisal of music (as in the sense that it is 'faithful to the original', whether this is in the performance or the technical reproduction). In the moral sense, fidelity may be used to describe both the character of a person and the actions that follow from it. Thus it might also be regarded as a moral quality.

In professional practice the notion of fidelity appears in various ways. It can be used to refer to the quality of being 'faithful to a vocation or professional calling', shown by the practitioner who acts in ways that display the virtues that are widely associated with that profession. In Koehn's (1994) terms this also includes those who pursue the values that define a profession as their primary objective. For allied health, medicine and nursing this is 'health', for teachers this is 'education', for social workers and youth workers it is 'social well-being' (which might include health in many contexts) and so on. Fidelity here means 'faithfulness to professional purpose'.

Another related quality is 'promise keeping', when the practitioner adheres to undertakings made to service users. Keeping one's word is highly valued across many cultures as a virtue. It is part of developing and maintaining *trust* and *integrity*. In many aspects of the work of the people professions, these qualities or virtues provide the basis for relationships between practitioners and service users that combine functional effectiveness with ethics. When it is not possible to keep a promise, from this perspective the practitioner has a *responsibility* to explain to the service user why this is so. There may be many good reasons why a statement made with good intent cannot be implemented, but this does not take away that responsibility, which reflects *respect* for the service user as a person. Such a possibility is encountered frequently in practice but may be dealt with differently based on whether the practitioner recognizes that it is an ethical matter. This is an example of why ethics cannot be considered as an optional extra that is only of relevance to those members of the people professions who are interested in the topic.

KEY TEXTS

- Beauchamp, T.L. and Childress, J.F. (2009) *Principles of Biomedical Ethics*. 6th edn (New York: Oxford University Press), Chapter 8 especially, pp. 311–322
- Botes, A. (1999) 'Nursing Ethics in a Developing Country', *Curationis*, 22 (1): pp. 64–67
- Crigger, N.J. (2010) 'Towards Understanding the Nature of Conflict of Interest and Its Application to the Discipline of nursing', *Nursing Philosophy*, 10 (4): pp. 253–262

freedom

SEE ALSO **autonomy; deontology; ethical egoism; human rights; liberalism; responsibility**

From many ethical perspectives freedom is a core aspect of what it is to be human. This concept is very closely associated with *autonomy* and *liberalism* and so, in different ways, of, *utilitarianism, deontology* and *human rights*. Two different forms of freedom are widely understood – 'negative' freedom or 'freedom from' and 'positive' freedom or 'freedom to'.

Negative freedom can be described as the state in which people are not subject to constraint in their actions. At one extreme this includes the ascription to imprisonment of 'loss of freedom'. However, in most situations negative freedom is understood to relate to the social barriers that might be placed in someone's way to proceed with an action. Examples might include laws, organizational policies and rules, the expectations of others where loss of co-operation or approval is seen as an impediment.

Being denied the necessary material resources to act is also an obstacle, so that 'freedom from poverty' is a commonly held application of this idea. Indeed, that freedom of this kind is regarded as good from many points of view suggest that not only is the state of poverty in itself considered bad but also the effect of poverty on the opportunities for people to act in the world define the way in which poverty is bad. For Nussbaum (2000), in her discussion of human capability, a core aspect of being human is to be able to make choices about how we live that are appropriate to our culture and context. Poverty often prevents people from participating in their community and can be seen as bad for this reason as much as because it also impacts on people's *dignity*, their health and so on.

Conversely, positive freedom can be described as the situation in which people have the capacity to act. This goes beyond the lack of impediments and should be considered as those things that people have from their circumstances that enable them to act. Such conditions can be divided into those that are 'natural' and those that are 'non-natural'. Natural freedoms include individual physical health and strength. However, it is also possible to argue that there is very little in the natural world that provides positive freedom in and of itself; rather, the way in which the natural world is acted on and organized is social and therefore should be seen as non-natural. For example, living in a geographical region that has many resources may present the potential for positive freedom, but agriculture and fishing are activities that in all but the simplest societies are socially organized. Therefore the freedom to obtain good nutrition is affected by social norms and customs, which in modern industrial societies include laws and policies, opportunities for employment and so on. Even the freedom to enjoy fulfilling relationships depends in part on the person's psychological, emotional and spiritual state that can be affected by the actions of others, as much as a relationship in itself partly depends on the actions of others.

There are many ways in which freedom from and freedom to can be seen as complementary. For example, freedom from censorship is also freedom to express one's opinions (free speech). Similarly, there are many states of freedom which can also be seen as freedom to live a fulfilling life, such as fear, abuse, illness and so on. However, *political* perspectives on ethics differ greatly in the way in which they approach freedom. The liberal position tends to give great weight to the concept of negative freedom. Freedom from constraint, in this sense is what liberty means. For many of the various strands that comprise liberalism, specifying what people might do with freedom from constraint would be seen as introducing new constraints. In contrast, a socialist perspective might suggest that it is not only possible but also necessary to specify what positive freedoms should be valued. The reason for this is that for some people to have greater freedoms from poverty, for example, may require other people to have actions constrained (being required to pay tax to pay for social welfare is an example of this). This understanding is grounded in the non-natural understanding of the origins of poverty, or whatever constraint from which people are to be freed, which in turn needs to be addressed socially.

One example of the way in which these views affect the people professions can be found in family and domestic violence. In most societies, including Western societies until very recently, this issue was widely regarded as a private matter between members of families. However, the view that increasingly prevails is that this constitutes a violation of the freedom of family members, most usually women and children, to live with freedom from fear and from injury. In order for this to be achieved it is necessary to limit the freedom of others, in this case mostly men, to express their thoughts and emotions in particular ways; for example, they may be prevented from expressing emotions through aggression and violence. A liberal perspective on this balance of freedoms emphasizes the use of law, with the main professional response therefore being to make available to the victims of such violence laws to protect their freedom from assault or threat. For relational- and community-based perspective this does not go far enough, because of the socially structured way in which such issues arise. From this perspective it is necessary to intervene more actively and provide women and children, and men when they are victims, not only with legal protections but also with services such as refuges, access to options for living away from the perpetrator or removal of the perpetrator from a home, physical health care and counselling, and to engage in public education about this as a problem. These different perspectives have quite divergent implications for law, policy and professional practices, including the use of tax-funded resources to provide such assistance to victims. For those liberals who regard taxation as a breach of negative freedom this presents a particular difficulty. Other liberals find more common ground with those who take a more interventionist approach because they recognize the way in which the exercise of *responsibility* is another key aspect of freedom, so that denying another person freedom from fear or assault then may reasonably have implications for the perpetrator's own freedom from constraint.

KEY TEXTS

- Epright, M.C. (2010) 'Coercing Future Freedom: Consent and Capacities for Autonomous Choice', *Journal of Law, Medicine and Ethics*, 38 (4): pp. 799–806
- Johnstone, M.-J. (2011) 'Choice and Human Freedom', *Australian Nursing Journal*, 19 (3): p. 22
- Ross, E. (2008) 'The Intersection of Cultural Practices and Ethics in a Rights Based Society: The Implications for South African Social Workers', *International Social Work*, 51 (3): pp. 384–395

futility

SEE ALSO beneficence; consent; consequentialism; non-maleficence; principles

A concept that has its origins in biomedical ethics, futility is a *consequential* principle. In that sense it may also be seen as a second order or subsidiary notion that defines a particular view of the outcomes of particular professional actions. Quite simply, the concept of futility is that an action which has no plausible chance of success should be regarded as bad or wrong. There are two main possible reasons why this may be so.

First, futile intervention is likely to cause harm to the service user. This may be actual physical injury, such as in the case of a medical or nursing procedure. Any pain or discomfort that is experienced by the service user could under such circumstances be considered as unnecessary, so that what in other situations would be accepted as part of receiving help becomes a problem. For the practitioner under these conditions it is then important to ask whether there is a moral *responsibility* to avoid such an act. For some practitioners it may be sufficient to ensure that the person has given their explicit informed *consent*. The exercise of *autonomy* could be thought of as taking preference over the opinion that the intervention has very little or no likelihood of success. For others, it may be considered a *duty* to emphasize to the service user that success is highly unlikely and so to actively try to dissuade any request to go ahead anyway. Given the *power* exercised by professionals this can be seen as effective, but reliance on persuasion depends on whether the service users understand and agree. In some situations, therefore professionals may well find that they may face the choice of refusing to act in particular ways.

Resolving decisions about interventions with little or no likelihood of success by dissuading service users through the way in which information is presented may be considered as *paternalistic*. However, making sure that people who may be in a vulnerable situation receive all possible information about the options that are available may be overwhelming, so it is very difficult for the practitioner not to have some impact on how this is received and understood. The final decision about whether to pursue an intervention that the practitioner considers futile will therefore involve a fine balance of judgement between these factors.

Second, futile intervention also may be considered to be an inappropriate use of scarce resources. Very few professional services have costs low enough for this to play no part in any consideration of their value. Whether interventions are paid for by the service user as a fee or are subsidized in some way from public funding the consumption of such resources for no good purpose raises ethical problems from the *utilitarian* perspective. The balance of human well-being is not appropriately addressed if resources that could used for something else (by the service user) or for other service users (if publicly funded) are taken up in actions that have little or no chance of succeeding.

Especially in services that are provided on a direct fee basis, there is an additional related problem of *over servicing*. For this reason, if practitioners are to take seriously the demands of both duty-based and consequential ethics, the wish to maximize income must be balanced with the claims of responsibility not to provide interventions that have no or little chance of success. Many professional bodies contain clear instructions to their members on this point within *codes of ethics*. In some circumstances of potential futility this may be sufficient, combined with the legal and business ethic of 'buyer beware', while in other areas of practice regulation by the wider professional community is helpful.

However, in all of these concerns, it is important to remember that any professional intervention has only a proportional chance of success. While in those supported by strong evidence this may be close to 100 per cent it can never fully reach that degree of certainty and there are also many areas in which all professions act where lower proportions are realistic. How low this likelihood can go before an intervention is considered futile is then a matter of judgement, of the individual practitioner in the specific content of an individual situation but this must be sustained by the wider professional community and evaluated against the continuing development of knowledge and skill in the field.

KEY TEXTS

- Beauchamp, T.L. and Childress, J.F. (2009) *Principles of Biomedical Ethics*. 6th edn (New York: Oxford University Press), Chapter 5 especially, pp. 166–172
- Thompson, R.J. (2011) 'Medical Futility: A Commonly Used and Potentially Abused Idea on Medical Ethics', *British Journal of Hospital Medicine*, 72 (?): pp. 969–969
- Trossman, S. (2011) 'Issues Up Close: The Practice of Ethics', *American Nurse Today*, 6 (11): pp. 32–33

h

harmony

SEE ALSO care (ethics of); Indigenous ethics; religion and ethics; ubuntu

Recognition of harmony as a value tends to be found in non-Western ethical systems, those of *Africa*, Asia and *Indigenous* or First Nations peoples. Across these various cultures and societies, there is a strong emphasis on a view that balance in the world is a primary good. Thus, harmony can be seen as a balance between all the different aspects of the world. This includes within one's self, between individuals, within families and communities, between human beings and other animals, between society and the physical world and between the physical and metaphysical (or spiritual) dimensions of reality. In each case, this balance is understood to be the *responsibility* of human beings, in that both as individuals and as groups it is human activity that can disturb the balance of the world.

For example, Hinman (2012) describes the Navajo *religious* concept of 'Holy Wind' as 'an ethic of harmony' (p. 67). This is not a formal theoretical system, but rather a culturally grounded practical way of considering what is good and right in human action relative to the relationships between people and between people and the world around them. The Holy Wind is seen as the source of guidance for human behaviour, with some similarities to the notion of 'conscience' – that is, it portrays an awareness of what is good and right that serves to advise each person on their actions. This is not a model in which people lack *autonomy* but is a way of describing the character of the person who does the right thing; this person is one who listens to the Holy Wind. Such a person is *virtuous*, in Navajo terms seen as 'one who lacks faults' (p. 65).

Confucian 'harmony' is described by Lai (2006, p. 157) as achieved through the recognition of status and appropriate relationships, as well as in *loyalty*. This frequently requires acquiescence to the way that things are supposed to be (shared established social norms). The goal is mutuality, with cohesive relationships that benefit everyone who is involved. Confucianism, in particular, emphasizes that these goals are achieved through the promotion of certain other key values, including *compassion* (grounded in recognition of common humanity), mutual responsibilities and reciprocity. Similarly, Daoism also points to acquiescence, although here it is because the goal is to seek contentment and peace within oneself. The Daoist approach is described by Lai (p. 168) as one that embraces conflict as necessary for human development and so harmony from this perspective comes from the acceptance of simplicity and diversity and is different to Confucianism. Thus, the sense that there is a single Chinese approach to ethics, let alone a unitary 'Asian ethics', has to be questioned. Nevertheless, there is common ground in seeking to understand and act on the value of harmony that separates these traditions from much of modern Western moral philosophy.

In African thought, the value of harmony is closely related to the notion of the 'unity' between people (Graham, 2002). Thus it is linked to concepts such as *ma'at* (rightness in the world) and *ubuntu* (identity through community) both of which emphasize balance between a person and the social, physical and spiritual context and as the heart of morality. In particular, Graham (2002, pp. 81–82) connects ma'at with the *ethics of care* as it expresses the value of relationships and recognizes women's perspectives on the world as central to ethical thought. Elders likewise have a central place in ma'at as they form a link between the generations that are part of the same families and communities (p. 83).

Because of the dominance of Western moral philosophy in formal professional ethics, the concept of harmony usually does not appear in *codes* and similar documents. Moreover, because of the emphasis in Western thought on notions such as autonomy as the basis for respect for persons and on the individual as the primary focus of morality, community- and relationship-based approaches have not had a great deal of impact. Similarly, perspectives such as *human rights* and *social justice* (understood from this Western standpoint) have tended to regard claims to the value of harmony quite critically, because of the association with the notion of acquiescence.

Thus it can be rejected as being a way in which those who are disadvantaged or who have less opportunity to exercise power can be oppressed, by being made responsible for ensuring harmony through 'giving in' to that disadvantage and oppression. However, both Graham (2002) and Lai (2006) reject this view and assert that if understood correctly the value of harmony is intertwined with justice in much the same way that proponents of the ethics of care argue for care (see, e.g. Kittay, 1999). In other words, when someone acting badly and wanting to avoid being called to account relies on an expectation that others will not dissent because this will be seen as unharmonious, they are acting unjustly. It is not only those who are in subordinate social roles who are expected to maintain harmony by focusing on their responsibilities but also those in more powerful or authoritative positions, perhaps even more so the latter.

For professionals, understanding these different views can be seen as important in working with service users whose cultural background emphasizes harmony as a primary value. The approaches that might be employed in cases where people expect to use conflict to challenge injustice may well not be successful if service users consider harmony to be primary as both a means and an end. For example, might it be more important to a person that harmony is maintained than that they overtly challenge something that is considered unjust? In health, it may be that an individual defers to wider family views about treatment because they value the reciprocal emotional and psychological support they receive in a harmonious group. Similarly, social workers, teachers and youth workers may find young people being expected to give priority to family or community group expectations in order to maintain harmony, in which the young people consider adhering to the group to be the good action even if this seems to be against her or his wants or interests.

This also raises questions for practitioners themselves, concerning their understanding of their own backgrounds and the values that they bring to their practice. To some extent, many practitioners may make decisions based on the maintenance of harmonious relationships, whether these are personal or professional. Finally, it should not always be assumed that service users and professionals from Western backgrounds do not themselves seek harmony. For example, in situations of family conflict, it is as likely that Western service users' preference would be for harmony to be restored as to pursue more abstract understandings of rights or justice. In all these situations what should be born in mind is that harmony does not have to be contradictory to rights or justice, but may often have a close resemblance in outcomes. The difference is in how these goals are pursued.

KEY TEXTS

- Davis, A.J. and Konishi, E. (2007) 'Whistleblowing in Japan', *Nursing Ethics*, 14 (2): pp. 194–202
- Epstein, I. (2009) 'Promoting Harmony Where There Is Commonly Conflict', *Social Work in Health Care*, 48 (3): pp. 216–231
- Hodge, D.R. *et al.* (2009) 'Moving from Colonization to Balance and Harmony: A Native American Perspective on Wellness', *Social Work*, 54 (3): pp. 211 219
- Konishi, E. *et al.* (2009) 'The Japanese Value of Harmony and Nursing Ethics', *Nursing Ethics*, 16 (5): pp. 625–636

honesty

SEE ALSO discourse ethics; fidelity; trust; truth; virtue

Often regarded as a *virtue*, honesty can be seen simply as *truth* telling. The honest person is the one whose words and actions match reality. However, in his discussion of *discourse* ethics, the German philosopher and sociologist Habermas (1990) draws distinctions between different ways of understanding truth in terms of (1) factual correctness, (2) normative rightness and (3) personal truthfulness. From this it might be argued that it is difficult to take a simple view of honesty as 'telling it like it is,' because only the first type of truth, factual accuracy, might be regarded as objective. There is a degree of objectivity about norms, in that these can be shared and discussed. However, when it comes to a personal understanding of the world, the third type of truth, personal truthfulness, must be seen as subjective.

From this it might be said that the honest person is one who seeks to communicate clearly in all three areas. They seek to be factually accurate, normatively right and subjectively truthful. Yet there are problems in achieving this. In Western legal systems, the idea of specifying 'the truth, the whole truth and nothing but the truth' is a phrase that is widely known. It raises the question of whether people are honest if they do not tell everything, or if they say not only what they know to be correct and right but also add things of which they are not sure. Both withholding aspects of what is known or believed or adding something that is not known or believed can affect the way in which other people understand communication.

The practical problems involved in honest communication and action include the possibility that service users may not accept, or be able to accept, all that needs to be said in order to be completely honest. So some practitioners may consider it to be necessary to provide information and ideas in stages, for people to be able to have the time to make sense of what is being said before they receive further information. If a practitioner decides to do this, because the responses of service users indicate that immediate full disclosure would be resisted or harmful, then careful communication is required to ensure that withholding information for a time does not then lead to distortions in what is heard and understood. In making this decision, the practitioner must also address the problem of *paternalism* explicitly, making such a choice carefully and as part of a process of truth telling. This is a *consequential* approach in that it seeks to base moral choices on the goal of the best possible outcomes for service users.

In terms of virtue ethics, honesty also includes intention. Seen from this perspective, a person who is mistaken in their communication but intends to tell the truth could be seen as honest. Indeed, the notion of 'an honest mistake' is used popularly to cover such an eventuality. In this sense, honesty is closely related to personal or subjective truthfulness. The way in which people view each other in this regard is based on their own observations: does the other person's actions match their words; do the other person's action and words match the hearer's own experience and so on? In this way honesty as a virtue is closely intertwined with *trust*. That is, to what extent can one person rely on another person's statements and actions as the basis for her or his own thoughts and actions? Trust is identified by many writers on professional ethics (such as Koehn, 1994; Tschudin, 2003; Beauchamp and Childress, 2009; Banks, 2012) as central to relationships between service users and professionals. The tasks of the people professions require that service users are also honest about their problems, their circumstances and other aspects of their lives, and this does not occur well if there is no trust in the practitioner.

Perceptions of honesty also have implications for *respect* between people. From a *deontological* point of view, if a person is not honest, then she or he is effectively not treating others as moral beings and at the same time they are not treating her or himself as a moral being either. One of the commonly used examples of the deontological principle of universalizability of the basis for one's actions is that it is impossible to generalize the claim to normative rightness in telling lies. That is, within this approach, if I say that it is acceptable for me to tell lies, then my claim has to apply to everyone else as well; I cannot make myself an exception without denying everyone else their humanity. In a world in which it is acceptable for everyone to tell lies then human relationships effectively become impossible because we cannot act together without confidence in each other's communication. Such an understanding also supports the importance of trust between service users and practitioners, for which the practitioner has considerable responsibility.

Honesty is widely understood as a primary value, whether sustained by any one major ethical approach or by a plural understanding of their combined implications. Practitioners share this common morality with service users and because it is part of everyday life it may often be assumed and only addressed explicitly when problems occur. In such situations, however, it helps to be aware of the issues and the ways in which being honest can require careful attention.

KEY TEXTS

- Begley, A.M. (2008) 'Truth-telling, Honesty and Compassion: A Virtue-Based Exploration of a Dilemma in Practice', *International Journal of Nursing Practice*, 14 (5): pp. 336–341
- Mayville, K.L. (2011) 'Technology, Cheating, Ethics, and Strategies for Creating a Culture of Honesty', *Chart*, 109 (3): pp. 6–10
- North, C.E. (2011)' Embracing Honesty', *Teaching Education*, 20 (2): pp. 125–132
- Sykes, R.L. (2004) 'Ethical Attributes and Professional Skills Development', *The New Social Worker*, 11 (2): pp. 4–5

honour

SEE ALSO **dignity; harmony; respect; virtue**

As with *harmony*, the value of honour is not widely addressed in formal professional ethics. Although it has some similarities with *respect*, there are also some important, if subtle, differences. Both describe the element of moral regard that can be present in the relationships between people. A person can be honoured and respected; indeed, it is good to be treated in this way by one's friends and neighbours. At the same time, these concepts also attach to the character and actions of the person who may be regarded as honourable or respectable. Thus, in more complex terms, these notions describe valued characteristics of the person, as these are perceived to draw out particular responses from others.

In addition, as with respect, honour is an aspect of the person's moral identity. However, it is here that the two ideas can be said to part company. The person who is dishonoured has suffered a different harm to the one who is disrespected. While disrespect attaches to the relationship between people in a given set of actions, to dishonour someone is to harm their moral identity more generally and deeply. Such a distinction can be seen in this way: honour is the ascription of goodness to a person, while respect recognizes the moral fact of their humanity. In other words, respecting humanity does not make any finer moral judgement than recognizing what it is to be human. In contrast, to dishonour someone is to attack the public acknowledgement of her or his goodness.

In this sense, honour can be understood as a form of *virtue* ethics. MacIntyre (1998, pp. 27–28, 57–58) relates it not only to Plato but also to Aristotle, noting that people value honour precisely because it is an external indication that others acknowledge their virtue. For Aristotle, virtue is the primary good, while for Plato, honour concerns the capacity of a person to engage in social relationships, such as having 'standing' in the community. As such, honours stands very close to the notion of *integrity*. It is in this latter sense that the notion of honour is usually understood in many different (non-Western) cultural contexts. There is also a widely shared focus on the way in which dishonour can be considered equal to disgrace. In turn, this latter concept involves the idea of shame, which is the feeling of disgrace within the person who is dishonoured. In some cultures where honour operates in this way, a person can be dishonoured by others who reflect her or his identity, such as family members, while in other contexts it is the actual person who attracts these judgements.

One example of the way in which honour may affect relationships between service users and professionals is in questions of privacy and *confidentiality*. The human problems with which the people professions are concerned are often matters about which people feel their moral identity is exposed to scrutiny. Not only things such as issues of poverty, the breakdown family relationships, problematic behaviour of children, addictions, crime and so on, but also problems of physical and mental health may be sources of embarrassment or shame. For this reason, taking care of privacy and confidentiality is not only about contractual and legal obligations but also about the morality of identity. As this can vary between cultures, it is important to recognize this in listening carefully to service users and their families.

Honour, therefore, has particular significance in the context of any given culture. For some, it may be the source of the problems brought to professionals for help, or it may affect how practitioners see their relationships with each other as well as with service users. This suggests that in multi-cultural contexts, practitioners need to be aware of this value and how it is integrated into the moral framework of everyday life for service users and colleagues alike. For example, in some cultures, it may be dishonourable for a woman to be spoken to by a man to whom she is not related. In this case, such an act both shames the woman by spoiling her social identity as a good person and also insults her and her family by implying that they are not good people. In such circumstances, it will be very hard to provide professional help unless a woman professional is available (Gilligan and Akhtar, 2006). In situations of grave danger to someone's life, male professionals may regard other values as having greater priority, but they might normally be expected to negotiate this with the individual and her family.

KEY TEXTS

- Aube, N. (2011) 'Ethical Challenges for Psychologists Doing Humanitarian Work', *Canadian Psychologist*, 52 (3): pp. 225–229

- Gilligan, P. and Akhtar, S. (2006) 'Cultural Barriers in the Disclosure of Child Sexual Abuse in Asian Communities: Listening to What Women Say', *British Journal of Social Work*, 36 (8): pp. 1361–1377
- Good, H. (2004) 'Honor Role', *Teacher Magazine*, 16 (2): pp. 46–48
- Peleg, R. (2008) 'Is Truth a Supreme Value?' *Journal of Medical Ethics*, 34 (5): pp. 325–326

human agency (includes self-determination)

SEE ALSO autonomy; deontology; freedom; human rights; responsibility

A core dimension of modern Western ethics is the idea that what it is to be human centres on *freedom* to exercise reason and to act in the world of one's own volition. Thus, for example, coercion (where someone is forced to act in ways that are against her or his will either by physical force or through social and psychological means) is regarded as bad or wrong, even at times as an *evil* because it destroys the very nature of what it is to be human. Both *deontology* and *utilitarianism* regard the human person as a moral agent in this way. Moreover, when that person is free to exercise agency, she or he can also be held morally *responsible* for her or his acts. This understanding of moral action is centred on the choices of each individual, assuming sufficient liberty for each person. For this reason, the set of ideas describing the way in which the world should be organized to make this possible is called *liberalism*.

Other perspectives may also regard the person as a moral agent. Indeed, the notion of responsibility can be seen in *African*, Asian and *Indigenous* ethics. However, in these approaches, the human agent is not considered firstly as a separate *autonomous* individual but rather as in relationship with family and community. This does not remove the ascription of agency from humanity; instead it places this within the networks of social relationships that make up everyday life. Thus, although Western liberal views of the individual lend themselves to formulation as categorical statements in *codes of ethics*, for example, the relational view is realized in everyday thoughts and actions.

There are two crucial ethical implications for interventive professions arising from the view of the person as a moral agent. The first of these is the very strong principles that unless the informed *consent* of the person is obtained to engage in a particular intervention the practitioner is violating that person's humanity. Without consent, even if the practitioner's actions are for the good of the service user, based on the professional assessment of needs and appropriate responses, then in moral terms the service user is being treated as an object rather than a subject. Only in life-threatening circumstances, where the person in need is unable to give or withhold consent, might it be said that there is a clear moral responsibility on the part of the professional to act without gaining consent.

Actions by professionals that ignore or over-ride human agency have come to be defined as a major ethical problem since the World War of 1939–1945. Under Nazism, medical doctors, nurses and other health professionals, social workers and teachers all participated in carrying out research on prisoners in concentration camps as well as other types of professional actions (Johnstone, 1994). This included inflicting pain, discomfort, *indignity*, distress and suffering on large numbers of people, almost always leading to their death. However, Hinman (2012, pp. 172–174) notes that moral change can be slow and such experimentation continued in countries such as the United States up to the 1970s.

The practice of informed consent, in which the practitioner is expected to explain an intervention and obtain the agreement of the person before starting to act, has become widely accepted as the best way to prevent such moral outrages. It also prevents less extreme harms that, nevertheless, violate the sense of the person as a moral agent. In the practices of community work, social work and youth work, this may be interpreted to mean that service users should always be involved in the identification of problems and of ways to deal with these problems, as well as in taking an active role in resolving them. The only limitations for this approach are the requirements of law.

Second, following from this, human agency requires that professional actions also address other ethical principles, including *fidelity*, *honesty*, *trust* and *truth*. While these can be considered as virtues, reflecting the moral character of the practitioner, their realization in practice also recognizes and responds to the moral identity of the service user as an agent. From a deontological perspective by embodying these virtues, the practitioner treats the service user as a moral end in her or himself and, at the same time, acts in such a way that the principle behind the action can be generalized to all people. Thus this basis for action not only reflects well on the practitioner but also embodies values that inform the way in which it might be expected the practitioner would wish to be treated by others.

There is, however, a perception among some practitioners of a problem in how this notion may be applied to children and also adults who have impairments in cognition or communication. To what extent is it reasonable to treat as a human agent a person who in other respects is not regarded within the wider society as fully 'competent' in this moral sense? Part of the concern here is that unless the person can be regarded as capable of forming a minimal understanding of that to which she or he is being asked to give consent then to ascribe agency to them is to place too great a burden on them, or even disingenuous because it takes as consent what is as likely to be a different reaction such as trying to please an authority figure. Of course, many ordinary people may act in this way (as the Milgram and Stanford psychology experiments demonstrated), but this is not normally taken to remove any sense of human agency when these people meet criteria such as age and lack of impairments to cognition or communication.

KEY TEXTS

- Clifford, D. and Burke, B. (2009) *Anti-Oppressive Ethics and Values in Social Work* (Basingstoke: Palgrave Macmillan), Chapter 3
- Le Granse, M. *et al.* (2006) 'Promoting Autonomy of the Client with Persistent Mental Illness', *Occupational Therapy International*, 13 (3): pp. 142–159
- Scheyett, A. *et al.* (2009) 'Autonomy and the Use of Directive Intervention in the Treatment of Individuals with Serious Mental Illnesses', *Social Work in Mental Health*, 7 (4): pp. 283–306
- Smith, K.R. (20) 'Psychotherapy as Applied Science or Moral Praxis', *Journal of Theoretical and Philosophical Psychology*, 29 (1): pp. 34–46

human rights

SEE ALSO **deontology; dignity; freedom; human agency; liberalism; politics**

Hinman (2012, p. 187) argues that 'the language of rights proved to be the most powerful language for moral change in the twentieth century.' In other words, although people may disagree as to what precisely constitutes 'a right', they are agreed widely across different national and cultural contexts that the idea of rights is extremely important in considerations of human conduct collectively as well as individually. This idea has been the foundation for major change in international law, the practice of governments and quasi-governmental bodies such as the United Nations, as well as individuals and collectivities such as professions.

Many discussion of human rights centre on the *Universal Declaration of Human Rights*, which was first made by the United Nations in 1948. (This was one of its first major acts following its formation.) The Declaration contains 30 articles that specify the basis of rights and state what rights are to be regarded as universal. The principles that underpin the *Declaration* are grounded in a view of what it is to be human. In other words, without these conditions being met, a person's life can be considered as less than 'truly human'. The values that support these statements include *freedom, dignity, human agency* and *moral equality*.

The association of these ideas with *deontology*, in particular the individualism of its approach, has formed the basis of criticism that the *Declaration* is a Western document. These ideas are stated in the United States and French constitutions; however, they also appear in the constitutions of countries such as Vietnam, because of the way in which Marxism as well as *liberalism* is based on such an understanding of what it is to be human. This is also the case for many other non-Western countries. This claim of cultural bias was also rebutted by Kofi Annan as General Secretary of the United Nations, when he said that 'It is never the people who complain of human rights as a Western, or Northern, imposition. It is too often their leaders who do so' (Annan, 1997).

Arguments about rights assume that these attach to the claims that people have on others. Rights 'holders' are those who can say that they have 'entitlements' to act or to have others act in certain ways. Thus, like freedom, there are both negative and positive rights. The first is an entitlement not to have something done to the person, or to be required to do something; the other is the entitlement to have something done or to be able to do something. From this, other people stand in relation to rights holders as duty bearers. These are the people who have (in negative rights terms) an obligation either not to prevent someone from acting or requiring them to act, or (in positive rights terms) an obligation to perform an act or to assist the rights holder in doing so.

Human rights can be claimed at all social levels, from the actions of governments towards whole populations to individuals' actions towards other individuals. The implication for practice in the people professions can be found at all levels. At the governmental level, members of these professions have an interest and may be actively involved in policy formation and implementation. Consequently, whether policies address human rights issues will be important. Similarly, at the community and personal levels, professions may well require their members to observe human rights. Actions that conflict with human dignity and agency will do so. It is not only respecting claims such as the right to life that might constitute a problem for the human rights argument, but also less obvious questions where difficult decisions may be required. Thus, for example, it is not only ignoring a service user's wishes or interests that constitute a breach of that person's rights. Using undue pressure or deceit to force a person to give consent to an intervention may also be considered such a breach. This can happen in practices such as obtaining consent to a surgical procedure, or to receive medication, gaining acceptance for a move from the service user's own home into a group care facility (such as a residential care or nursing home) and in persuading a parent to accept the removal of a child or children to a place of safety such as a foster family. In each instance, great skill is required from practitioners in ensuring that in observing human rights that people are *respected* in these types of situations.

One aspect of human rights that can be problematic for some practitioners is the view of human rights as a *political* matter. This is based on the question of whether professions ought to be considered as separate from politics. However, not only does politics affect the matters that concern the people professions (children and families, communities, education, health, people with disabilities, older people, and so on) but there are also some political acts such as torture and terrorism that members of professions may sometime be expected to be involved in and against which practitioners need to have safeguards. Indeed, it was precisely these sorts of questions that led the World Medical Association (WMA, 1964) to produce the landmark *Helsinki Declaration*, which has set the terms of such debates ever since.

The particular notion of 'right to life' causes some ethical debate for professions in health in particular, especially as technology has become more complex and sophisticated. It is now possible to maintain a person's physical functioning beyond the point at which it can be said that there is evidence for their mental functioning, or indeed to the point where physical functioning is dependent entirely on artificial means. From some perspectives, decisions to withdraw life support in such a situation can be seen as making a deliberate choice to end a person's life and so breaching their right to life; alternatively the notion of this right in such circumstances in regarded by others as qualified or non-existent. Similarly, the right to abortion that is now widely accepted in many Western and other advanced industrial countries is not uniformly approved by all ethical positions. From some perspectives such a right is tangible and absolute, while others argue that it is a breach of the right to life of the foetus. As with the withdrawal of life support, such arguments about the way in which the idea of human rights is interpreted for these questions tend to be resolved using other ethical approaches, either deontological or *consequential*.

Professions' *codes of ethics* and related documents frequently contain statements that require members to observe the rights of service users and other fellow citizens. For example, at the international level, this applies to medicine (WMA, 2006), occupational therapy (WFOT, 2006), nursing (ICN, 2006) and social work (IFSW/IASSW, 2004), with many of their member country associations also making reference to this idea. Others, for example, psychology (IUPS, 2008), address respect for human dignity as a primary value and, while not citing human rights directly, provide references or links to human rights materials, such as the *Universal Declaration*. Therefore, human rights as a principle can be seen as very important across the professions.

KEY TEXTS
- Gauthier, J. (2009) 'Ethical Principles and Human Rights: Building a Better World Globally', *Counselling Psychology Quarterly*, 22 (1): pp. 25–32
- Ife, J. (2012) *Human Rights and Social Work*. 3rd edn (Melbourne: Cambridge University Press)

- Pavlish, C. *et al.* (2012) 'Health and Human Rights Advocacy: Perspectives from a Rwandan Refugee Camp', *Nursing Ethics*, 19 (4): pp. 538–549
- UN (1948) *The Universal Declaration of Human Rights* (New York: United Nations) – accessible at http://www.un.org/en/documents/udhr/> (this version is in English, with many other language versions available)

i

Indigenous (First Nations) ethics

SEE ALSO autonomy; harmony; human rights; justice; oppression; respect

Identification of specific 'ethics' of Indigenous or First Nations peoples is difficult, because of the wide diversity between the various cultures whose history of colonization now links them. These notably include Australia, Canada, Greenland, New Zealand, some of the Pacific Islands and the United States, although there are also many other countries where communities can be considered as Indigenous (UN, 2007). Nevertheless, there are some broad commonalities of core social values that provide the basis for considering Indigenous people as a distinct grouping in this sense (as might be done through the notions of *African*, Asian or Western values and ethics). It is this understanding that informs the United Nations (2007) *Declaration on the Rights of Indigenous People*.

One of the important commonalities of this kind is the strong relationship between people and land in Indigenous cultures (UN, 2007). This can be expressed in terms of sayings such as 'we do not own the land, the land owns us' or the notion that each generation has a *responsibility* to care for the land and to live in *harmony* with it. It is from this basis that values and beliefs about right human relationships and actions are drawn. Similarly, Indigenous cultures tend to place great emphasis on right relationships between human beings and other animals, plants and so on. Indigenous cultures have not traditionally had the sorts of formally structured systems of moral philosophy that have underpinned ethics in many other parts of the world, including Europe, Asia and parts of Africa. The values and beliefs of Indigenous people are found in lore, or laws. Consequently, colonizers tended over a very long period of time not to recognize that these are highly developed systems of morality that share many points of comparison. For example, different Indigenous ethics variously contain principles of *care*, *dignity*, *integrity*, *justice*, and *respect*, among many others, that are found in the more formalized systems of values in other parts of the world, although they may be expressed in many different ways and explained using different terms.

It is in this context that the tendency for community to be a central feature of Indigenous values and beliefs must be understood. As with the ethics of Africa and Asia, Indigenous peoples mostly consider human identity to be grounded in group membership, such as of families, clans or groups of clans (that using European concepts are often now understood as 'nations'). It is on this that responsibilities and obligations are based, structured around social roles such as that of 'elder' in addition to those of biological family. For this reason, the notion of family in Indigenous societies is slightly different from that in the colonizing cultures as it can be expansive and based on values that either did not traditionally exist or have faded in the latter through processes of modernization. This can be problematic for formal professional systems, in which expectations about the way that wider family members are involved in decision-making and care provision can be based on majority culture family structures. This can led to conflict over who should be allowed to participate in such matters or to misunderstandings about people's roles. In parts of the world such as Australia, Canada, New Zealand and the United States, it has led in the past to practices that are now recognized as discriminatory and as having harmed whole communities across several generations.

The understanding of values concerning both land and family is important for the practices of the professions. In all of the countries with histories of being colonized, Indigenous peoples share a common experience of drastically worse outcomes for child well-being, education, health and other aspects of social welfare. Therefore Indigenous people, although often small minorities in these societies, are found disproportionately among the service users of the people professions. This presents practitioners with considerable ethical challenges in that to act on their professional values, such as *human rights* or social justice, logically requires attention to the values and beliefs of Indigenous people (as stated in the *Declaration on the Rights of Indigenous Peoples* of 2007). Yet, so far as the application of universal values does not accommodate Indigenous perspectives, then Indigenous values must be addressed over and above universal values. It is this principle that lies behind the idea of affirmative action and that makes the different treatment of people in an ethnic minority position something to be pursued rather than a form of discrimination to be avoided (Kymlicka, 1989).

KEY TEXTS
- Bennett, B. *et al.* (2012) *Our Voices* (Basingstoke: Palgrave Macmillan)
- McCleland, A. (2011) 'Culturally Safe Nursing Research: Exploring the Use of an Indigenous Research Methodology From an Indigenous Researcher's Perspective', *Journal of Transcultural Nursing*, 22 (4): pp. 362–367
- Tupara, H. (2011) 'Ethics, Kawa and the Constitution: Transforming the System of Ethical Review in Aotearoa New Zealand', *Cambridge Quarterly of Healthcare Ethics*, 20 (3): pp. 367–379
- Weaver, H.N. (2002) 'Perspectives on Wellness: Journeys on the Red Road', *Journal of Sociology and Social Welfare*, 24 (1): pp. 5–15

informed consent

SEE consent

integrity

SEE ALSO **fidelity; honesty; loyalty; trust; truth; virtue**

Many writers, both moral philosophers and members of the people professions, see integrity as one of the most important *virtues* (Tschudin, 2003; Beauchamp and Childress, 2009; Sercombe, 2010; Banks, 2012; Hinman, 2012). It implies the integration of the moral character of a person, the way in which the various qualities combine to comprise the person. Thus it conveys a sense of ethical wholeness or completeness. From this, it can be said that integrity is the drawing together of virtues such as *compassion, courage, fairness, fidelity, honesty, loyalty, respect, trust* and *truth*.

There is no agreement between commentators on precisely which of these qualities are required for integrity; nor does all discussion identify all of them. What is common to various understandings of integrity in professional ethics is that it can be seen in characteristics such as *competence*, consistency, humility, impartiality, patience and reliability (some of which may also themselves be regarded as virtues). Beauchamp and Childress (2009, p. 42) also discuss integrity in terms of its opposites, which they consider are exemplified by 'hypocrisy, insincerity, bad faith and self-deception'. Thus, integrity is about the way in which a person achieves ethical wholeness.

An example of integrity discussed by Beauchamp and Childress (2009, p. 43) is that of a practitioner who refuses to participate in an intervention or procedure that she or he considers breaches other strongly held moral principles. In the health context, such situations may arise both in decisions about providing certain treatments or in withdrawing treatment. In social service contexts, likewise, decisions to do or not to do certain things can cause practitioners ethical concerns because of the way in which strongly held values impact on the way interventions are or are not undertaken. In both cases, such moral concerns can be independent of questions about the possible effect of interventions. Indeed, they usually are, in that if a treatment or an intervention is regarded as unlikely to be beneficial (it is or is most likely to be *futile*) then other ethical considerations would be brought to bear on such a decision.

One of the biggest challenges to integrity for members of the people professions is the extent to which their practices occur within organizations. Acting on integrity can place the practitioner in conflict with the organization where they work. Many professional practitioners regard themselves as working 'for' the service user, but to do this most allied health professionals, nurses, social workers, teachers and youth workers, as well as many medical practitioners, are employed by service providers such as hospitals and clinics, non-government community organizations, social-welfare agencies and schools. The practitioner who either insists on acting or refuses to act because she or he is not willing to compromise deeply held beliefs and values can place themselves in conflict with others who also consider that they have a moral claim on the practitioner's commitment, loyalty and so on. In some instances, these potential conflicts are avoided because organizations themselves have *codes of ethics* or of conduct that are grounded in widely help professional values. The emergence of managerialism in education, health and social welfare in recent years has impacted on this, in that professional values may sometimes be in conflict with organizational values. Where there are established ethical mechanisms, such as ethics committees, these can assist in such instances. However, there are also many organizations that rely on managerial authority in decision-making and under such conditions practising with integrity may at times require clarity, courage and self-understanding; it may also be helped by humility, openness and trust on all sides.

KEY TEXTS

- Banks, S. (2012) *Ethics and Values in Social Work*. 4th edn (Basingstoke: Palgrave Macmillan), Chapters 2 and 3
- Begley, A.M. (2008) 'Truth-Telling, Honesty and Compassion: A Virtue-Based Exploration of a Dilemma in Practice', *International Journal of Nursing Practice*, 14 (5): pp. 336–341
- Tschudin, V. (2003) *Ethics in Nursing: The Caring Relationship*. 3rd edn (Oxford: Butterworth-Heinemann)

j

justice (includes distributive, retributive and restorative justice)

SEE ALSO equality; fairness; social justice

The moral philosopher Hinman (2012, p. 221) offers a particular interpretation of the ancient Greek view of justice, which underpinned the teaching of Socrates (469–399 BCE) and Plato (429–347 BCE). Justice is *harmony* both within the person and between people in a society. In this way of looking at the notion, justice is both a *virtue* and a *principle* that together form two parts of a whole. To sustain the virtue of justice, Hinman states, the just individual must live in a just society. Likewise, the just society has to be composed of just individuals. Another way of understanding this relationship between the inner states of people and their outward membership of a society is through the idea of balance. In Western countries, justice is often portrayed in an ancient Greek figure of a woman holding a sword in one hand (representing authority to judge), scales in the other (representing balanced judgement) and wearing a blindfold (representing a stance of impartiality or *fairness*). Where the idea of harmony suggests complex networks of human relationships that of balance portrayed in this way indicates more abstract, formal principles.

In modern philosophy, the main problem with the platonic notion is that it could be possible to see a slave-owning society as just if it was harmonious, as indeed Plato did of his own society in ancient Greece. This clearly is incompatible with the concept of *human rights* and its related concepts and principles. Lai's (2006, pp. 78–79) consideration of the same ideas in Confucian thought points to a different way of distinguishing these competing understandings. She argues for separating justice as a way of describing a particular type of personal state or set of social relationships (which can be described as 'normative' because they establish what should be seen as the norm of character and action) and as a way of thinking about such qualities, states and actions (what is technically known as a 'meta-ethical' approach, which is a set of overarching ethical ideas). This helps to identify two important ways that the notion of justice is used in discussions about formalized professional ethics and the values and actions of individual practitioners.

Another very important distinction to draw between different uses of the idea of justice, whether as harmony or balance, is that of 'distributive' justice as compared to 'retributive' justice (and other ideas that follow from that, such as 'compensatory' and 'restorative' justice). There is also a connecting idea, that of 'desert', whether a particular circumstance or outcome is 'deserved', that informs thinking about both of these types of justice.

To take distributive justice first, this notion refers to the balance in the spread of resources, opportunities, rewards and other ways that people obtain what is seen as necessary to live a decent human life. Such resources can be physical, financial, social, relational or a combination of these. For example, the way in which a society is ordered can limit opportunities to gain or access to such resources to some people on the basis of particular social characteristics. These can include 'race', culture and ethnicity (e.g. members of ethnic minority groups), sex (women and girls), sexuality (people who are not heterosexual), disability (people who have physical or mental incapacities) and age (people who are very young or very old). This understanding of justice is sometimes also known as *social justice* (and is addressed in a separate section of this book).

One of the most influential approaches to the distributive idea of justice in the modern era is that of John Rawls (1921–2002 CE). Rawls argues that justice is best understood as a balance of opportunity to access those things that are needed to live a human life. This rests on two sub-principles: that the greatest possible *freedom* is available to everyone (limited only by the impact of one person's freedom on that of another); and that any *inequalities* should in some way be to the advantage of those who are least well off and open to everyone. Rawls also argued that this way of judging what is just would be agreed by all reasonable people if they had to choose without knowing what life opportunities they would end up with. This complex idea can be seen more clearly in reverse by considering the case of someone who does not think that socially funded provision for people with severe disabilities is fair because they have to pay tax and asking if that person or someone they care about has a disability and insufficient resources to live as normal a life as possible. Rawls' concept suggests this is not a just position to hold and that a society organized on this basis would not be just.

Historically all the professions that are the focus of this book have, at least at times, been concerned with distributive justice. For example, this can be seen in work done to create and sustain the provision of education, health and social welfare for disadvantaged individuals, families and communities. For some professions, such as social work and youth work, this is often seen as a major focus of their work stemming from their origins in the nineteenth century (CE). Others, such as allied health, medicine, nursing and school teaching, are not necessarily so widely concerned with this question, although they do have strong traditions of addressing problems both of access to education, health and social welfare and of the ways in which disadvantage and injustice create problems in the first place. In many parts of the world, and at various times in the history of the twentieth century (CE) in Western countries, these professions have worked together to develop practices and advocate for policies that will challenge such injustices. This may also have an international dimension, with the involvement of these professions in humanitarian, aid and development work.

Retributive justice concerns the way in which societies respond to someone who has done something to harm another person. This may include punishments or exacting compensation to compensate for the damage or loss caused by the act in question. The significance of this type of justice for the people professions is usually in the way that they interact as professions with the justice system. For example, members of all of these professions may be employed in the provision of education, health and social welfare to prisoners, or may be involved in providing justice services to people who are regarded as having offended but are not imprisoned, such as in community corrections or probation. Such roles, however, may create ethical challenges for practitioners. For example, the core idea of *fidelity* that the first *loyalty* of the professional is to the service user may not fit easily with such contexts. Practice in the justice system is likely to require that the professional participate in systems that are intended to form a punishment of some kind and in such situations there are limits to the loyalty to the service user that can be realized. In Western countries in recent years, professions increasingly set limits on what is regarded as acceptable for a member to do, such as in the involvement of medical practitioners and nurses in judicial executions where this is still practised. International ethical statements may give some basis for practitioners in other parts of the world to opt out of such activities (see IFSW/IASSW, 2004; ICN, 2006; WMA, 2006), but these are not easily enforced and individual practitioners may themselves consider the demands of a legal system to be acceptable in this regard and so choose to participate.

One alternative to orthodox retributive justice that has become more widely recognized recently is that of restorative justice. The principle in this is wrong acts disturb the balance of social relationships, which may also be thought of in terms of harmony. Justice in this sense is then achieved by restoring that balance or harmony. The practice that follows from this is for the person who is seen as having acted wrongly to make amends by performing some positive act, which may include apologizing to the victim or undertaking some practical tasks such as mending or replacing property that has been damaged or lost. This approach originates in *Indigenous* ethics, particularly from the Maori traditions in New Zealand. Its use has involved psychologists, social workers, teachers and youth workers who seek to provide positive ways of assisting both offenders and the communities of which they are part. It models the underlying idea in that it incorporates balance between the interest and needs of offenders and victims.

A notion that connects the ideas of distributive and retributive justice is that of 'desert'. Some positions with regard to distributive justice might see imbalances of life opportunities and access to resources as a *consequence* of choice made by individuals and communities. The notion of 'the deserving poor' influenced ethical thought in early social work, for example. Similarly, practitioners in health may not consider the needs of someone as compelling if they have caused their own injury or problem. Likewise, in retributive justice the receipt of punishment is widely regarded as 'what that person deserves'. These are widely held beliefs and to the extent that professional practitioners share them it is because they are members of their societies. However, as the professions' ethics have developed through the twentieth century (CE), this has increasingly come to be seen as problematic. Debates around this raise the question of *responsibility*. In the social welfare field, emphasis now tends to be placed on the connections between poverty and disadvantage and crime, for example. Consequently considerations of desert of this kind are widely thought to be open to question. In contrast, in health the problem of desert in the sense of taking an individual's actions into account are more likely to be resolved through a *utilitarian* view that looks at the likely benefits from the use of scarce resources to treat someone who may then recreate the problem through their behaviour and so waste the resource that could have been used for someone else.

KEY TEXTS

- Beauchamp, T.L. and Childress, J.F. (2009) *Principles of Biomedical Ethics*. 6th edn (New York: Oxford University Press), Chapter 7
- Edwards, I. *et al.* (2011) 'New Perspectives on the Theory of Justice: Implications for Physical Therapy Ethics and Clinical Practice', *Physical Therapy*, 91 (11): pp. 1642–1652
- Orme, J. (2002) 'Social Work: Gender, Care and Justice', *British Journal of Social Work*, 32 (6): pp. 799–814
- van Hooft, S. (2011) 'Caring, Objectivity and Justice: An Integrative View', *Nursing Ethics*, 18 (2): pp. 149–160

1

liberalism

SEE ALSO autonomy; deontology; freedom; human rights;
universalism; utilitarianism

Probably the most influential philosophical idea to emerge from the
processes of modernization in Europe from the sixteenth century
(CE) onwards is that of the moral and political *freedom* of the individual. This perspective asserts that the primary good is found in
the achievement of the maximum possible liberty for each person;
hence it is called liberalism. It is this idea that has been the origin
of debates about *human rights*, as well as modern interpretations of
consequential ethics in the particular approach of *utilitarianism* and
also of *deontology*.

The foundational concerns of liberalism lie as much in politics
as they do in ethics as this is popularly understood. The work of
philosophers such as Thomas Hobbes (1588–1679 CE) and John
Locke (1632–1704 CE) sought to address societies that were moving
rapidly from structures in which monarchs held considerable,
if not absolute, power and the position of most people was as a
means to the achievement of the ruler's ends, to use those ethical
terms, to a world in which each person was to be seen as an ethical
end in themselves. From this view, the modern interpretations of
notions such as *autonomy, human agency, respect* and *responsibility*
have developed, as well as the more detailed or subsidiary principles
such as *confidentiality* and *consent*.

The modern view of professions and of professional ethics in
many ways can be seen as a liberal phenomenon. It is not only that
the predominant view of ethics that is reflected in the statements
of the international peak bodies are grounded in liberal concepts,
although this is the case (e.g. see IFSW/IASSW, 2004; ICN, 2006;
WMA, 2006), but also that the very idea of formalized *codes of ethics*

itself stems from the abstract rationality that defines the way in which such statements are constructed. It is on this basis that codifying moral requirements becomes possible.

The liberal world in which professional ethics have become formalized in this way is one of relationships between strangers, or at least of people whose primary relationship is that of service users and practitioner, and not of people who are family and neighbours sharing many or all aspects of life. Indeed, when people do share many such aspects of life, as happens for example in rural practice in highly developed countries, this can be experienced as ethically challenging because the usual approaches to ethics assume separation of roles.

Exceptions to this idea can be seen in the work of teachers and also of allied health, nursing and social work practitioners who provide sustained personal care, such as in residential services. In these situations, practice requires that personal relationships are formed, which necessarily cannot be contained within the sorts of boundaries that make sense in urban contexts or in roles where service use and practitioner only meet with respect to the particular issue or problem. There are some elements of the liberal perspective that continue to be important, such as *impartiality* (each person has the same significance), but in these situations such a principle is better understood through the *ethics of care* as a matter of balancing the unique relationships and commitments that the practitioner may have with each service user. However, as with the rural practitioner, the nature of the professional role means that genuine friendships, which by definition are partial (people differ in their significance), present ethical difficulties that have to be managed very carefully.

It is also for these reasons that liberalism tends to be regarded by some non-Western critics as inherently culturally biased. For example, *Confucian ethics* (including the notion of filial piety), *African* perspectives such as *ma'at* and *ubuntu* and *Indigenous ethics* all emphasize the moral identity of the person as a member of collectivities, such as families and communities, as much as or prior to the person's identity as an autonomous individual. It is this difference that lies at the heart of ethical consideration of working 'across' or 'between' cultures. For example, the practitioner working from a liberal perspective, and whose understanding of ethics is informed by liberalism, may encounter the expectations of a service user from a different cultural background as a challenge if the service user expects family and community elder to be involved in discussions about their situation. Negotiating confidentiality in such a situation, for example, can create a moral hazard for the practitioner, while for the service user it may be encountered as being unhelpful or even obstructive.

This cultural dimension to the way in which liberalism defines professional ethics has particular implications for multi-cultural societies. For example, if liberal values are to be varied according to cultural background, who should decide which values can be rethought? How should someone's cultural identity be perceived and who decides? Indeed, underlying all of these questions, is it reasonable to treat people differently on grounds of culture or is this discrimination (Kymlicka, 1989)? What does different recognition suggest for the question of human rights and the treatment of all people as morally equal on the grounds that they are human (as in deontology). All of these questions point to the basic problem that liberalism is a *universal* position. That is, it argues that the same values apply universally, to all people equally. Against this, philosophers such as Iris Marion Young (1949–2006 CE) have argued that it is not possible to treat people equally by treating them all the same, because this ignores their unique characteristics and so inevitably takes some values as the standard that actually apply more to some people than to others. This is the argument for positive affirmation, in which equality of respect is achieved by valuing difference.

In practice, some degree of interpretation of liberalism occurs, as practitioners seek to address the individuality of the service users with whom they are working. Ways around different views of who should know what and be involved in decision making can reconcile a liberal and a family or community focused understanding by seeking to grasp clearly what the primary service user or service users wish for themselves. This does not mean that practicalities have to be ignored, nor the reasonable requirements of professional ethics, but that compromises can be negotiated. It should also be noted that cultures are not static and that liberal perspectives are increasingly informing values in non-Western contexts as societies industrialize and become more complex. For this reason assumptions cannot be made in individual situations and to respond effectively practitioners need to develop their capacities to work interculturally.

KEY TEXTS

- Brown, M.B. (2011) 'Three Ways to Politicize Bioethics', *American Journal of Bioethics*, 9 (2): pp. 42–53
- DeFillipis, J. (2009) 'What's Left in the Community? Oppositional Politics in Contemporary Practice', *Community Development Journal*, 44 (1): pp. 38–52
- Gostin, L.O. (2004) 'Health of the People: The Highest Law?' *Journal of Law, Medicine and Ethics*, 32 (3): pp. 509–515
- Young, I.M. (1990) *Justice and the Politics of Difference* (Princeton, NJ: Princeton University Press)

loyalty

SEE ALSO **fidelity; trust; virtue**

Loyalty may be understood as a person maintaining her or his commitment to another person or people, so that these others can depend on the person. This is a *virtue*, which can be summed up in the phrase, 'I knew I could rely on her to stick with me in this matter.' Loyalty is more than a matter of reliability, although that is part of it, because it also implies that the loyal person chooses to support the other even when this may not be convenient or easy.

Beauchamp and Childress (2009, p. 311) connect loyalty with *fidelity*, that is, faithfulness to serving the interests of service users. In many situations, this can mean pursuing what is right for the service user even if this means the practitioner puts the service user's interests ahead of their own and of others. Yet they also note that in practice loyalty is problematic. First, in reality it is very hard for any practitioner to achieve this degree of commitment to a particular service user (whether this is an individual person or a group such as a family or a community). All service users should be able to expect that professional helpers will consider their needs and interests. So, in response to this, practitioners balance their loyalties between all those who are looking to them for assistance. For this reason, it may be said that a type of *utilitarianism* becomes inevitable, even while the practitioner is in general committed equally to each of her or his service users. Quite simply, with limited time and other resources, some choices must be made and loyalty does not provide a sufficient basis to do this.

Second, it is possible to understand loyalty to require a practitioner to go 'beyond the call of duty'. As Beauchamp and Childress (2009, p. 311) note, for a practitioner to demonstrate that degree of commitment may be 'praiseworthy', but if this goes beyond what the community might normally regard as defining good practice, then this is too high a standard to set as a professional ethic that could apply to everyone. Such a choice would be called *supererogatory*, that is, 'above expectation'. (This is discussed in more detail in a separate section of this book.) Loyalty to one's friends, by contrast, would have a very high threshold by comparison.

Third, practitioners have to resolve competing loyalties not only between various service users but also between service users and colleagues or employing organizations. As Beauchamp and Childress also note (2009, pp. 313–314), the status and roles of professions affects the extent to which the idea of loyalty to service users may be the source of ethical challenges. Their example is that of nursing, as the health profession that is most defined by the decisions of another profession (medicine); allied health and social work, by comparison, have a degree of autonomy in forming their own assessments (compare with Tschudin, 2003; Sercombe, 2010; Banks, 2012). However, some allied health professions, nursing and social work, along with youth work, share an ethical commitment to advocating for the interests of their service users that can at times bring them into conflict with colleagues or organizations. As with medicine and psychology, these professions may all at times have roles in which they exercise a statutory or an authoritative function with regard to service users on behalf of another entity, such as the state or a company. In such circumstances, loyalty to service users is likely to be understood in terms of doing what is necessary while at the same time avoiding harm (the principle of *non-maleficence*). An example of such a situation is that of mandatory reporting of suspected child ill-treatment, which now occurs in many developed countries. Here, the statutory requirement takes precedence, supported by notions of the best interests of the child outweighing those of the parents who is also a service user. Resolving all such challenges requires balancing loyalty with other ethical principles and concepts.

Finally, although professionals may experience loyalty on the part of the service users, this cannot be expected or assumed. Especially in a modern urban setting where relationships between service users and professionals are often not primary, basing an approach to practice on the expectation that service users will be, or even should be, loyal to professionals is morally risky. It is not only that the sort of *trust* that is necessary to sustain this type of loyalty has to be earned and sustained. More importantly, the moral concern for the professional should be for her or his own values, actions and ideas and not those of service users, unless they form a reasonable part of the focus of the help or intervention. In sum, the loyalty of service users may be enjoyed when it occurs but it cannot be expected as a *right*.

KEY TEXTS

- Beauchamp, T.L. and Childress, J.F. (2009) *Principles of Biomedical Ethics*. 6th edn (New York: Oxford University Press), Chapter 8
- Girod, J. and Beckman, A.W. (2005) 'Just Allocation and Team Loyalty: A New Virtue Ethic for Emergency Medicine', *Journal of Medical Ethics*, 31 (10): pp. 567–570
- Nojhof, A. *et al.* (2012) 'Professional and Institutional Morality: Building Ethics Programmes on the Dual Loyalty of Academic Professionals', *Ethics and Education*, 7 (1): pp. 91–109

m

ma'at

SEE ALSO harmony; Indigenous ethics; justice; principle; religion and ethics; respect

One of the major ideas that informs ethical thought in *Africa* is ma'at. While its origins lie in the ancient Kemetic (early Egyptian) culture of the Nile valley region of northeastern Africa, its influence stretches across Africa as a continent (Karenga, 2004). In the *religion* of this period, ma'at is portrayed as a goddess, while more generally, ma'at is a way of thinking about moral values.

Graham (2002, p. 70) describes ma'at as having a 'multiplicity of meanings', including 'truth, justice, propriety, harmony, balance, reciprocity and order'. These are to be understood as an interconnected group of *virtues*, each of which contributes to a moral whole. At the same time, ma'at can also be understood as a *principle* through which ways of organizing social relationships and institutions can be considered (Karenga, 2004, p. 3). Taken together, these two explanations show that ma'at can be thought of as an all-embracing moral philosophy that addresses every aspect of the world. Thus, there are many similarities with the developing moral thought in other parts of the Mediterranean and Middle Eastern regions of that period. Moreover, these ideas continue to be found throughout Africa (as they also have parallels clearly occurring in contemporary Asian and *Indigenous* moral thought).

Karenga (2004) emphasizes that ma'at is concerned with personal and social well-being together. In other words, it is not possible to separate concern with individuals from concern with families and communities. For example, duties and obligations within these relationships form a balance in which *care* and *justice* are interdependent, if they can be distinguished at all. It is for this reason that Karenga appears to come close at times to suggesting that reciprocity is the central value of ma'at, although he is clear that it embraces all the values noted above. Moreover, it is important to recognize that the understanding of justice here is relational, not legalistic. It is not that someone performs an act only out of expectation that the other person will then provide something in return, but rather out of recognition of a relationship of mutual co-operation. In turn, the performance of acts that express the values that comprise ma'at will promote right action in responses of others. Conversely, the person who does not express ma'at injures others and in turn is likely to suffer. Again, parallels can be drawn with the ancient Greek distinctions between virtue and vice, with notions of greed, lies, selfishness and so on exemplifying the opposite of ma'at.

Ma'at also has spiritual dimensions. These have not simply originated within a particular religious system, but over time have become disseminated within cultures that do not make a separation between the personal, social, ethical and spiritual. Although he does not address ma'at specifically, Mbiti (1990), an African theologian, refers to the values and concepts that others ascribe to ma'at in his description of the connections between the self, others and social institutions. Indeed, Mbiti's description of the central African world-view that, 'I am because we are; and since we are, therefore I am' (1990, p. 160) (which is an interpretation of the concept of *ubuntu*) can be seen as a summary of the shared human life. As Mbiti puts it,

> It is a deeply religious transaction. Only in terms of other people does the individual become conscious of his [sic] own being, his own duties, his privileges and responsibilities towards himself and towards other people. When he suffers he does not suffer alone but with the corporate group; when he rejoices he rejoices not alone but with his kinsmen, his neighbours and his relatives whether dead or living. (1990, p. 160)

In such a world-view, the reciprocity, balance and *harmony* that are important elements of ma'at are each part of the fabric of social relationships. They hold together the values of care, justice, *truth*, propriety and order. Furthermore, discussions of ma'at tend to agree that ma'at is not simply a system of concepts but must be practised: one does not 'think' ma'at, one 'does' ma'at.

For the people professions, assisting people for whom ma'at ideas and practices are the focus of morality means that attention will need to be given to understanding the broader personal and social implications of their beliefs. Ways of working with the idea of the person-in-community that is core to ma'at means that individualized of explanations of needs, problems and issues in education, health, social well-being and so on are unlikely to be satisfactory for service users. This can challenge dominant professional perspectives around privacy and *confidentiality*, and around assessment and diagnosis, as well as in the formulation and implementation of interventions (including medical treatment). Certainly, in some professions such as social work, there are arguments for the rejection of principles such as confidentiality as inherently and unhelpfully Eurocentric. (This is summarized in Graham, 2002.) People of other cultures may consider that it is right and good that information and decision making is shared among family members or senior members of a community. In this case, it is worth considering that the service user's own view of the world provides a reference point for making sound judgements about the way in which professional ideas may be understood and regarded. Indeed, the principle of *respect* for the person can provide a bridge between the moral implications of individualistic and collectivistic worldviews. The inclusion of family members (which itself raises questions about who counts as family) or community representatives in some aspects of professional practice can go against the strongly held values of contemporary people professions. Yet in other ways, the values that are part of professional ethics find strong resonance in the various dimensions of ma'at. For this reason, addressing ma'at in practice may require cultural sensitivity and a willingness to think flexibly, without clashing outright with professional ethics. Indeed, cultural sensitivity and flexibility can benefit many groups of people. This leads Graham (2002, p. 97), among others, to argue that by considering ma'at as part of the wider ethics of the people professions, practices with all people can benefit.

KEY TEXTS
• Graham, M. (2002) *Social Work and African-Centred World Views* (Birmingham: Venture Press), Chapter 4

- Karenga, M. (2004) *Maat: The Moral Ideal in Ancient Egypt: A Study in Classical African Ethics* (London: Routledge)
- Moodley, R. and Bertrand, M. (2011) 'Spirits of a Drum Beat: African Caribbean Traditional Healers and Their Healing Practices in Toronto', *International Journal of Health Promotion and Education*, 49 (3): pp. 79–89

moral fluency

SEE ALSO codes of ethics; discourse ethics; responsibility; wisdom

Many practitioners and others think of ethics as a set of principles that have to be applied; often, this will be expected to take the form of a *code of ethics*. While this approach can be sufficient as a framework for formalizing ideas about ethics, it suggests that such principles can be considered as 'rules to be followed'. An alternative perspective is to regard ethics as part of the practice skills of the professional. For example, Sellman (1996) proposes the notion of 'moral fluency', arguing that practitioners should develop the capacity to incorporate ethics into their everyday practice for themselves in much the same way that they develop skills and strategies. In this sense, ethics is not something to be learned as an external set of rules or principles but should be internalized as an ongoing reflective process in which practitioners consider their own actions, thoughts and feelings and engage in dialogue across their profession and beyond.

In a similar vein, Husband (1995) argues for the 'morally active practitioner'. This embodies a view of ethics as grounded in the notion of *responsibility*, as opposed to the 'reasoned and legitimated set of externally prescriptive guidelines, backed by the coercive pressures of a regulatory body' that comprise formal professional codes of ethics (p. 87). Here, then, we have a contrast between acting on the basis of ethical *duty* and being morally responsible. Even if one is guided by the *deontological* understanding that an act becomes morally worthy because it is performed for reasons of duty (as opposed, say, to the pleasure given by doing the right thing for Husband), it is not possible to distinguish such an act from mere habit or conformity.

These concepts face a significant problem in the everyday world of professional practice. While it is possible for the private practitioner, or a member of a partnership or collective structure, to exercise the sort of moral fluency or responsibility being suggested by these critiques, for the very large number of practitioners who are employed by organizations, whether government, third sector (non-governmental and not-for profit) or privately owned, the scope of the professional role is based on a primary relationship with their employer. Under these conditions, it is even possible for decisions to be based entirely on technical judgement, no matter how complex or fine-grained this may be. There is, therefore, a risk that ethics likewise comes to be treated as a technical matter.

Yet, as both Sellman (1996) and Husband (1995) note, the foundations of professional ethics also offer ways in which practitioners can grasp and engage with moral reflection. Ideas such as responsibility are interwoven with notions of duty and of *care*, requiring that consideration be given to the balance between *principles* and *consequences*. The implication, which Husband addresses explicitly, is a *pluralist* view of ethics in which moral issues are never settled 'once and for all' or by reference to one overarching principle that is capable of resolving all debates.

To be morally fluent and active requires that practitioners are consciously aware of the ethical dimension to their work. In turn, this demands that each practitioner should develop her or his capacity to understand, think about, debate and rethink the ethics of practice. This is the capacity that is known as *wisdom* or, to use the technical term, *phronesis*. It is not that each practitioner must become a moral philosopher, but rather that ethics is too important to be left to ethicists to hand out instructions. This argument points to the way in which responsibility has to be taken by each practitioner in the context of their membership of their professional community.

KEY TEXTS

- Husband, C. (1995) 'The Morally Active Practitioner and the Ethics of Anti-Racist Social Work' in R. Hugman and D. Smith (eds), *Ethical Issues in Social Work* (London: Routledge)
- Sellman, D. (1996) 'Why Teach Ethics to Nurses?' *Nurse Education Today*, 16 (1): pp. 44–48
- Stevens, P. (2000) 'The Ethics of Being Ethical', *The Family Journal: Counseling and Therapy for Couples and Families*, 8 (2): pp. 177–178

n

non-maleficence (non-malfeasance)

SEE ALSO beneficence; care (duty of); principles; responsibility

Possibly the oldest recognized professional ethic is that which is often attributed to Hippocrates (*circa* 460–377 BCE): 'first do no harm'. (This is sometimes rendered as, 'above all else seek to do no harm'.) Hippocrates is often credited with being the forerunner of Western medicine. In addition to developing an understanding of the human body that is not very different from modern ideas, he also appears to have practised and taught in ways that still make sense as a model of the 'good physician'. Whether he actually stated this principle in these terms, it now bears his name.

Beauchamp and Childress (2009, pp. 149–150) note that non-maleficence is sometimes regarded as a subset of *beneficence* (seeking to do good). Referring to the work of the moral philosopher Frankena (1973), they distinguish between the *principle* 'not inflicting evil or harm' from those of 'seeking actively to prevent harm', 'removing evil or harm' and 'promoting the good'. The latter three principles Beauchamp and Childress regard as elements of beneficence. Understood in this way, the key aspect of non-maleficence is in intentionally refraining from acting in a way that causes harm. As they go on to argue, this principle can then be divided into three dimensions: acts concerning the *duty of care* that a practitioner can be said to have towards a service user; non-intervention (both withholding and withdrawing intervention) and distinctions between what is intended and what may be foreseen but not intended.

Breaching duty of care can be synonymous with failing to observe the requirements of non-maleficence. Certainly, lack of attention to one's professional *responsibilities* must fail the test of seeking not to do harm. Non-maleficence implies more than the luck of not causing harm but that the practitioner should actively address her or his attention to this goal. Thus, if harm is caused even though all reasonable steps were taken to prevent it, the practitioner has conformed to this ethical principle. There is a *consequential* or *utilitarian* aspect to this principle, insofar as the balance of good over bad outcomes may be used to evaluate professional action. For example, a bruise caused by a nurse in giving an injection may be unavoidable while safeguarding a child from future illness, or in the longer term and with greater impact the distress resulting from the removal of a child from her or his family may be balanced against the protection of the child from abuse or neglect that is occurring.

Decisions to withhold or to withdraw interventions also raise questions about potential harm. Here too there is a balance between outcomes and intentions. What can reasonably be expected to result from such an action again is the standard by which it will be judged. *Futile* interventions are a clear case, although even in such circumstances there may be grounds to proceed in order to satisfy service users that everything possible has been done. Where the balance of benefit to harm from an intervention is less easy to predict, matters can become more complicated. In these cases, which are large in number, quick decisions by practitioners acting alone or just in collaboration with a single service user are best avoided. There is widespread support for the view that such decisions are better made in a shared way, involving service users with their families and others who they may wish to consult, as well as colleagues and wider professional networks. Practitioners in some settings, such as hospitals, may well have formal committees to assist in decision making to ensure that hasty or collusive actions are not taken to the harm of all involved. This can include end-of-life decisions, statutory interventions such as the removal of a child from a family and so on.

Beauchamp and Childress (2009) draw a distinction between what is intended in an action and what may be foreseeable but is not intended. That is, to decide if a bad outcome that results from an action intended to cause a good outcome is acceptable, it must be asked whether the bad is a deliberate means of achieving the good or simply an unfortunate side effect. This often is a fine distinction, as their example of different situations where judgements may be made about different circumstances involving abortion of a foetus in order to save the life of the pregnant mother. They conclude that the defensible argument here is that a known possibility of a bad outcome is only justified in the reasonable expectation of achieving an equally significant or greater benefit. So the position we can reach on abortions will then depend as much on how we view the relative moral weight of the life of the foetus as against the life of the mother.

Finally, Tschudin (2003, p. 64) notes that although obligations of beneficence are owed only to specific people (we do not have a responsibility to do good for anyone and everyone), those of non-maleficence are general. In other words, all actions, whether personal or professional, might reasonably have the aim not to harm anyone.

KEY TEXTS

- Beauchamp, T.L. and Childress, J.F. (2009) *Principles of Biomedical Ethics*. 6th edn (New York: Oxford University Press), Chapter 5
- de Vries, M.C. and Verhagen, A.A.E. (2008) 'The Case against Something That Is Not the Case', *American Journal of Bioethics*, 8 (11): pp. 29–31
- Tschudin, V. (2003) *Ethics in Nursing: The Caring Relationship*. 3rd edn (Oxford: Butterworth-Heinemann), Chapter 4

O

oppression (includes anti-oppressive values and action)

SEE ALSO human rights; justice; social justice; respect

The concept of oppression has become a major moral and political issue in professions such as social work and youth work, as well as among some allied health professionals (most notably occupational therapy), medical practitioners, nurses and teachers. It is grounded in an analysis of society that argues that opportunities to live a decent human life are not equally distributed. It shows that social advantage and disadvantage are distributed differently according to a person's sex, ethnic or 'racial' identity, religion, age, physical and mental abilities and health status, sexuality and geographical location. Thus oppression can take the form of sexism, racism, sectarianism, ageism and discrimination against people on grounds of ability or health, heterosexism and other forms of discrimination. These factors are seen as likely to affect life chances, most especially related to income and wealth, and from this to basic necessities such as water, food and adequate shelter, as well as access to education, health and social services. While the needs addressed by the people professions are not all necessarily caused by low income and other forms of disadvantage, some have these causes and all can be exacerbated by them. Therefore, oppression is to be seen as sets of social relationships and institutions that serve to create and maintain the unequal distribution of access to the means of achieving a good human life, to the benefit of some individuals and groups and the detriment of others.

For Clifford and Burke (2009), attention to oppression in professional ethics is a broad area for inquiry rather than a developed approach. They argue that thinking about the moral and political implications of recognizing oppression as an ethical issue inevitably draws on a range of approaches rather than being located within one specifically. Their view can be regarded as situated within the framework of ethical *pluralism* or the common morality perspective (for comparison, see Banks, 2006). This means that it seeks to bring together and to integrate aspects of thinking from *deontology, utilitarianism, virtues, justice, human rights* and the *ethics of care*. Arguments about why oppression is bad or wrong, and what professionals' *responsibilities* are in the face of it, necessarily draw on a range of these ideas together.

Examples of areas in which it may be argued that members of the people professions have such responsibilities include access to services. This in turn can be affected by the way in which problems and issues are perceived, how assessments and diagnoses are conducted, the way in which interventions are planned and implemented and so on. In each area of work, practitioners can recognize and address questions of discrimination and oppression. An instance can be seen in the way in which ethnic minority populations in Western (and some other) countries face greater health needs but often lack the financial and social resources to access appropriate help. Ensuring that all aspects of educational, health and social services provide appropriate responses, including both the practice of individuals and the policies and systems within which practice occurs are important ways in which this can be achieved. In the instance of ethnicity, this includes cultural sensitivity in interpersonal communication and the way in which interventions are conducted, it includes having interpretation available if needed, and it may require practitioners to be flexible in their thinking about things such as who constitutes family and the meaning of *respect* and *confidentiality*.

At the centre of questions about oppression and practices that oppose oppression are the principles of *non-maleficence* and *beneficence*. If the practices and service structures of the people professions contribute to oppression, then this can be seen as causing harm, which clearly violates the first of these two principles. From this it can be said that there is an obligation to seek changes that will prevent this from happening. Beyond this, however, the principle of beneficence can be seen as more restricted: non-maleficence is a general obligation and beneficence applies to those towards whom there are specific duties. Yet it can be said that the people who either already use or potentially will use these professional services are those towards whom there is this specific duty. Drawing particularly on notions of justice (which common morality balances with non-maleficence and beneficence), Young (1990) argues that affirmative action of this kind becomes a moral obligation precisely because such 'positive discrimination' (through attention to the specifics of people's social identities) opposes oppression and thus enables practices and policies to fulfil many other aspects of professional ethics.

KEY TEXTS

- Clifford, D. and Burke, B. (2009) *Anti-Oppressive Ethics and Values in Social Work* (Basingstoke: Palgrave Macmillan), Chapters 1 and 6
- Corneau, S. and Stergiopoulos, V. (2012) 'More Than Being against It: Anti-Racism and Anti-Oppression in Mental Health', *Journal of Transcultural Psychiatry*, 49 (2): pp. 261–282
- Dong, D. and Temple, B. (2011) 'Oppression: A Concept Analysis and Implications for Nursing and Nurses', *Nursing Forum*, 46 (3): pp. 169–176
- Epstein, M. (2011) 'If I Were a Rich Man Could I Sell a Pancreas? A Study in the Locus of Oppression', *Journal of Medical Ethics*, 37 (2): pp. 109–112

over servicing

SEE ALSO **fidelity; honesty; integrity; non-maleficence; trust; truth**

One of the risks of attentive responses to the needs of others is in the possibility of doing too much. When this occurs, it can be understood as 'over servicing'. There are two particular reasons why this can happen: concern not to do too little and possible gain for the practitioner in doing as much as possible.

First, in many highly developed countries, there are legally supported *human rights* for service users that give them avenues for redress if a practitioner fails to provide all the assistance that is possible. This may then lead practitioners to do more for service users than they might otherwise regard as necessary or even appropriate, out of a concern not to be seen as doing too little. More and more tests may be done, the conclusion of counselling or therapy postponed, cases are not closed despite reaching their goals and so on. Sometimes it is service users themselves who seek further intervention, perhaps because they do not accept that everything has been done and especially if their problem has not been resolved in the way that they expected. In other instances, it may be that individuals or agencies are reluctant to say that they can do no more out of a concern with possible legal implications. Such a situation is to be seen as 'defensive practice'.

However, to provide more assistance or treatment than is suggested by good assessments and supported by the best available evidence is to act in bad faith – that is, it breaches the *fidelity* of the relationship between the practitioner and the service user. This is still a serious ethical matter if the risks are otherwise negligible, because there is the moral harm of potentially deceiving service users and others by such an action. When other risks are greater, then the inappropriateness of over servicing also fails the test of *non-maleficence*.

In situations where a practitioner chooses to do more than is professionally indicated irrespective of the wishes of service user or without their knowledge, because she or he gains in some way, this is also a serious breach of ethical obligations. This is most likely to occur in situations where the service user pays a fee directly to the professional, or where fees are charged to a third party such as an insurance fund. It may also happen if a practitioner wishes to gain further experience with a particular type of practice, so that the service user unknowingly is used to meet the needs of the practitioner and not served for their own needs.

This second type of over servicing is highly problematic. It not only is based on *dishonesty*, but it also fails to treat the service user as an *autonomous* person and undermines their *human rights*. As with defensive practice, the primary focus is on the needs of the practitioner, but here it goes further because such actions effectively use other people as a means to ends to which they have not knowingly been a party. Furthermore, it cannot be justified on the grounds of *utility* as the balance of probable benefit lies very much in the favour of the practitioner. So, on this basis, such actions fail all possible tests in terms of the ideas on which professional ethics is founded.

KEY TEXTS
- Brameld, K.J. and Holman, C.D.J. (2005) 'The Use of End-Quintile Comparisons to Identify Under-Servicing of the Poor and Over-Servicing of the Rich: A Longitudinal Study Describing the Effect of Socioeconomic

Status on Healthcare', *BMC Health Services Research*, 5: p. 61 [accessed on 24/9/2012 from http://www.ncbi.nlm.nih.gov/pmc/articles/ PMC1236924/]

- Huong, D.B. *et al.* (2007) 'Rural Health Care in Vietnam and China: Conflict between Market Reforms and Social Need', *International Journal of Health Services*, 37 (3): pp. 555–572

P

partiality and impartiality

SEE ALSO care (ethics of); emotion; justice; universalism

The *liberal* approaches to ethics that tend to dominate professional ethics derive from attempts to create scientific systems of thought that matched the growing influence of scientific method in other areas of human inquiry. Both *deontology* and *utilitarianism* argue for a *universal* view, in which impartiality is regarded as a key element. Indeed, it can be said that one of the strengths of these positions is that they are intended to apply equally to everyone, simply on the basis of being human. So, for example, from a deontological perspective, a categorical imperative gains its moral force from the fact that it is universalizable: if I say that lying or stealing are acceptable, then I have to allow that this applies to everyone, I am not able simply to allow it for myself or my friends. Similarly, in utilitarianism the moral weight of each person is equal, with nobody favoured or left out: everybody counts for one and only for one. Even when circumstances are taken into account, the objective is that nobody should be disregarded, as in thinking about *justice* and *human rights*. In this way, thinking impartially about moral questions can be seen to express *fairness*. In a world that was struggling free from arbitrary absolute rule to one in which people could claim *freedom* to exercise moral judgement, as was the case in medieval Europe, this notion was extremely important.

Yet there are many situations in which the claims of impartiality appear to create other problems for thinking about ethics. For example, in non-Western cultures, it is often argued that family and community relationships are the cornerstone of morality. This can be seen in *African*, Asian and *Indigenous* ethical systems of thought. More recently in Western moral philosophy, there have been an increasing number of developments that also question the way in which this understanding of impartiality is inadequate. Williams (1981) famously used the hypothetical example of a man faced with a choice of rescuing only one of two people from the sea and argued that where one of these people is his spouse the fact of this relationship alone is morally sufficient to justify his choice to rescue her and not the other. If he is required to use moral philosophy to explain himself, says Williams, he is being expected to 'have on thought too many' (p. 18). It is such attachments that make us human. The *ethics of care* likewise challenges the standard liberal interpretations of impartiality.

However, those who wish to ensure that the morality of relationships is addressed in professional ethics do not seek to impose unlimited partiality in favour of a dehumanized view. Held (1993) and Tronto (1993), among others, have argued that the ethics of care is compatible with ethics of justice, where justice assumes that relationships do not become the sole criterion for moral judgement but take their place in a range of aspects. The assumption here is that in the public realm, the context from which classic liberal views of impartiality originate, injustices do not emerge because relationships are allowed to become the paramount value.

For example, to adapt William's illustration, it may well be the case that no one will blame the health professional who treats their own child ahead of others when the child is in a serious condition and needs immediate help. However, if their child's needs are less serious than others, different moral questions begin to be asked. Similarly, the school teacher who gives their own child additional guidance in their studies and does not offer other children the same opportunity cannot be regarded as acting badly if this is not occurring in the time that she or he is paid to teach the children in the school.

In this way, it can be seen that impartiality is a useful principle in a complex world where many relationships are with strangers. However, we also live in a world where we have close relationships with family, friends and neighbours. An ethical system that requires us to ignore these altogether does indeed seem to ask too much. For this reason, recent debates have sought to find better ways of balancing partiality and impartiality, giving significant value to close relationships while at the same time recognizing the importance of fairness and openness in the public realm.

KEY TEXTS

- Nortvedt, P. *et al.* (2011) 'The Ethics of Care: Role Obligation and Moderate Partiality in Health Care', *Nursing Ethics*, 18 (2): pp. 192–200
- Tronto, J. (1993) *Moral Boundaries: A Political Argument for an Ethics of Care* (New York: Routledge), Chapter 5
- Woodard, V. (1999) 'Achieving Moral Health Care: The Challenge of Patient Partiality', *Nursing Ethics*, 6 (5): pp. 390–398

paternalism

SEE ALSO autonomy; benevolence; human agency; human rights; power

Pellegrino and Thomasma (1988) regard the promotion of *autonomy* as the single most important aspect of *beneficence* in practice. That is, from their point of view, the best interests of the service user are achieved through achievement of her or his own preferences. This argument is made against a long-standing tradition, especially in medicine, of regarding beneficence as in conflict with autonomy and the service user's *right* to know about all aspects of her or his life. The letter includes the right to make decisions and give consent to or refuse interventions. Consequently, it also assumes the right to receive all relevant personal information, while at the same time being afforded confidentiality and privacy.

Paternalism represents the contrary view that beneficial action requires the professional practitioner to consider how much autonomy the service user is capable of exercising. In situations where the practitioner judges that the service user will be harmed by receiving information or being asked to state preferences, paternalism suggests that it is best for the professional to act without sharing information and decision making. This view rests on two assumptions. The first is that the professional practitioner possesses knowledge and skills, supported by the capacity for sound judgement based on experience, that are not possessed by the service user. The second is that in many, if not most circumstances, service users may suffer harm such as distress, confusion or despair if they know the full extent of the facts about their problems.

In relation to the first of these assumptions, it may be noted that the very nature of the professions means that practitioners do have access to knowledge and skills that are not held by others; they also have experience that others do not have. This is why people seek their assistance. However, this in itself does not take away the value of autonomy for service users, which strips people of their humanity. Against paternalism it can be argued that the implications of this are that practitioners have an obligation to provide information in a clear and understandable way, and to support service users in expressing their own preferences. In other words, the issue is usually how rather than whether information is provided and service users actively involved in decision making. This is what has become the norm in recent decades as the way of achieving beneficence.

In relation to the second point, it can be agreed that there are circumstances in which people may be harmed by being given information or expected to take *responsibility* for making decisions. For example, people whose cognitive functioning is impaired by serious mental ill-health or by the misuse of drugs may in certain conditions lack the capacity to exercise autonomy. In those circumstances, some arguments are made that a limited form of paternalism is appropriate, as beneficial action requires that people be protected from the worst implications of their lack of autonomous judgement. Mental health legislation in many countries is based on this position, which Beauchamp and Childress (2009, pp. 209–211) describe as 'soft paternalism'. For example, such legislation may *empower* professionals to require a person to receive treatment against their will when they are demonstrably threatening the life of another person or themselves. A distinction may be drawn here between someone threatening suicide and a person who is making a considered end-of-life decision to ask for the withdrawal of treatment.

One area in which professionals may also regard a degree of paternalism to be appropriate is in working with children and young people. Particularly school teachers and some youth workers and social workers have to resolve this in many aspects of their work. The assumption is that children and young people cannot be expected to take full moral responsibility for their decisions or actions. Indeed, the origin of the word 'paternalism' is in 'the authority of the father'. However, it is contrary to good educational theory to act as if children and young people lack all moral capacity (Carr, 2000; Sercombe, 2010). Rather, these professions seek to respond to their service users on the basis that they accord the maximum possible autonomy to young people, in relation to the age and capacity of those with whom they work. The goal of education and youth work can be expressed as the achievement of good moral development on the part of each young person as they move into adulthood. Thus, even with children and young people, at the most only a very soft view of paternalism is widely held.

KEY TEXTS

- Beauchamp, T.L. and Childress, J.F. (2009) *Principles of Biomedical Ethics*. 6th edn (New York: Oxford University Press), Chapter 6
- Bransford, C.L. (2011) 'Reconciling Paternalism and Empowerment in Clinical Practice: An Intersubjective Perspective', *Social Work*, 56 (1): pp. 36–42
- Zomorodi, M. and Foley, B.J. (2009) 'The Nature of Advocacy vs. Paternalism in Nursing: Clarifying the "Thin Line"', *Journal of Advanced Nursing*, 65 (8): pp. 1746–1752

phronesis (practical wisdom, prudence)

SEE ALSO **virtue; wisdom**

Knowledge of the *virtues* may assist in understanding the dimensions of the good character, but in itself is unable to provide a basis for choosing which virtues are appropriate to a given role or circumstances or even how to act in particular situation. Aristotle's (384–322 BCE) approach to the virtues centred on the concept of 'phronesis', which variously is translated as prudence or practical *wisdom*. What distinguishes phronesis or prudence from other ways of seeing wisdom is that it refers to the capacity to make wise judgments that are integrated with good actions.

For example, in the situation where a particular practitioner displays the virtue of *compassion*, this in itself will not be sufficient to guide actions. How does this practitioner know where to draw the line between compassion and pity on one side and callousness on the other? Too much feeling for another's plight, which is how pity may be understood, can lead to poor judgement insofar as the moral *responsibility* of the other becomes obscured; this, in turn, can lead to an inappropriate *paternalism* and lack of *autonomy* for the service user. The epithet of 'bleeding heart' or 'do-gooder' is sometimes attached to the person who is seen to make this mistake (although why a practitioner should wish to 'do bad' is never addressed in this criticism). On the other side, if insufficient compassion is shown, then the practitioner becomes callous. This can be seen where so much blame is attached to the choices made by service users that have contributed to their problems that practitioners become reluctant to provide assistance. Callousness exhibited by someone in the people professions can sometimes be an indication of 'compassion fatigue' or 'burnout' (Hugman, 2005, p. 54). Thus, the phronesis of compassion is in knowing the right balance between pity and callousness and being able to achieve it in everyday practice.

To some extent, therefore, prudence or practical wisdom can be regarded as a skill or capacity. This then raises the question of how it can be developed. Aristotle's answer is, first, that virtues do not occur one at a time (Hinman, 2012, p. 274). The virtuous practitioner is one who displays all the virtues of good practice to a sufficient degree. In this way, each virtue informs others, so that keeping the right balance helps the person to maintain and develop her or his moral character. Yet this still does not fully answer the question. It is also necessary to consider practical wisdom like any other practice, not only in the professions but also in a craft or trade, a sport, music or art. In other words, it is something that has to be developed through practice and reflection, in the manner suggested by the Socratic notion that the examined life is the only one worth living. It is the pursuit of practical wisdom that helps the practitioner to integrate the virtues and to continue to develop them through consciously considering them in practice (Bondi et al., 2011).

KEY TEXTS

- Bondi, L. et al. (eds) (2011) *Towards Professional Wisdom: Practical Deliberations in the People Professions* (Farnham: Ashgate)
- Sellman, D. (2009) 'Practical Wisdom in Health and Social Care: Teaching for Professional Phronesis', *Learning in Health and Social Care*, 8 (2): pp. 84–91
- Tsang, (2008) 'Kairos and Practice Wisdom in Social Work Practice', *European Journal of Social Work*, 11 (2): pp. 131–143

pluralism (including 'common morality')

SEE ALSO principles; relativism; universalism

The major approaches to ethics each make a distinct claim on the way in which we should regard what is good and right and how these are to be achieved. *Deontology, consequentialism* and *virtue* ethics each present a particular way of understanding and acting. Consequently, many arguments about ethics favour one or the other approach and some devote themselves entirely to showing how one approach is superior to the others in producing the best ideas and practices. Because each of these approaches, and the *principles* that are linked to them such as *human rights* and *justice*, are held to apply equally to all people, they should be understood as *universalist*. Against this, it is argued that what is good and right is related to particular social and cultural contexts or to ways of looking at ethics. This leads to arguments for cultural or ethical *relativism* (the differences between which are discussed in the relevant section of this book).

However, there are many moral philosophers and applied ethicists who regard such distinctions as unrealistic and unhelpful. Their argument is that there can be a legitimate range of ways in which the ethics of a particular situation can be addressed and that diverse values can be held in relation to the same question. The term pluralism derives from the way in which this approach seeks to hold together a plurality of values in a complicated but necessary tension. The development of this perspective is usually attributed to British philosopher Isaiah Berlin (1909–1997 CE), although he also drew on the work of American thinkers such as William James (1842–1910 CE) and John Dewey (1859–1952 CE). Berlin's argument is that the major traditions of moral and political philosophy tend to advance one value position, which he termed 'monism' (Berlin, 1969). Yet in everyday life people struggle to balance the competing demands of values that can be either incompatible (it appears that they cannot exist together) or incommensurable (literally, not able to be measured, but here meaning having no common standard of evaluation). For example, *liberty* may be inconsistent with *equality*, love and personal commitments with *fairness* or a preference for peacefulness with valuing a world in which there are small children. Values such as beauty, *fairness* and *truth* may even be difficult to compare, as they clearly do not share any comparative standards of evaluation. Not all of these values are moral, but they all relate to choices people make about the sort of world in which they wish to live.

More recent discussions of the pluralist position are provided by Kekes (1993) and Hinman (2012). Both argue for a way of thinking about the competing claims of values and ethics that do not rely on a fixed resolution by reference to one specific approach. As Hinman puts it, neither ethical relativism nor ethical monism can deal with all of the practical moral requirements of living in an increasingly diverse world (2008, p. 30). Pluralism, he asserts, is able to help us to understand others and to tolerate difference while still being able to say that something is *evil*. It also, at the same time, enables us to accept the possibility that we may be wrong. It seeks the balance between, on one side, being unable to act 'because it is all just different' and, on the other, moral arrogance. Thus, pluralism requires the openness and reflection of prudence (*phronesis*).

An example of the need for these qualities in ethical deliberation that is often encountered by practitioners is in relation to cultural differences. For example, although it can be argued that the differences between Western and other approaches to ethics may at times be exaggerated, the Western traditions of valuing one's parents clearly take different forms and often have a different impact to the Asian value of *filial piety*. One of the most contentious of such questions is the practice of female genital cutting called female genital mutilation and female circumcision, respectively, by its opponents and proponents. Arguments about abortion, euthanasia and so on also have cultural dimensions to them. These debates directly involve members of the people professions both as professional and as ordinary members of their societies. Consequently, there are wide variations in the values that practitioners bring to ethics debates. Some of these seek to find ways of achieving dialogue between cultural perspectives and other value differences, while others seek to defend the expression of different values.

Beauchamp and Childress (2009) argue that there is a 'common morality' that operates in everyday life. That is, because most people do not live with a strict monistic system of values, it is entirely plausible that professions should do likewise. They suggest that the three major approaches of deontology, virtues and consequentialism that are combined in this way. From this, they then propose four ethical principles: *respect* for persons (deontology); *beneficence* (virtue); *non-maleficence* (virtue) and justice (consequence). This approach has become widely influential, especially not only in the biomedical field for which it was first developed, but also in other professional areas as well (e.g., see Sercombe, 2010; Banks, 2012). The practical way of working across these different approaches requires that people listen to each other carefully, seek to find common ground and not simply to win the argument at all costs. For some people, this is too high a price – for example, the person who regards individual human rights as paramount will find it extremely difficult to allow any room to the argument for female genital cutting as this is almost always practised on young girls (where ethically there are problems of consent, the disadvantages faced by women in many societies and so on). Nevertheless, in a plural world it is also important for all points of view to be listened to. Pluralism and common morality approaches seek to do this, recognizing that agreement may not always be possible and certainly is unlikely to be permanent, but that by balancing the claims of different perspectives it is possible to find shared ground.

KEY TEXTS

- Hinman, L.M. (2012) *Ethics: A Pluralistic Approach to Moral Theory*. 5th edn (Boston, MA: Wadsworth), Chapter 2
- Hugman, R. (2013) *Culture, Values and Ethics in Social Work: Embracing Diversity* (London: Routledge), Chapter 6
- Nagel, T. (1979) *Mortal Questions* (Cambridge: Cambridge University Press), Chapter 8

politics

SEE ALSO **freedom; human rights; liberalism; oppression; social justice**

The people professions exist in societies where there are competing demands on resources as well as over the roles and functions of the professions. Debates about these occur both between the professions and the surrounding society and within the professions themselves. In this way, the people professions have to be seen as inevitably involved in politics. Certainly in the past and even today in many respects, the boundaries between moral and political philosophy have been either regarded as non-existent or at least as somewhat vague and difficult to define. Consequently, the same *principles* that can be used to consider the actions of one individual in relation to another (e.g., the practitioner and the service user) are also used to examine questions about the relationships between groups in a society and between nations.

The various systems of political thought, including *liberalism*, conservatism and socialism, each assert various values concerning the way in which people should live together in a society. For example, each of these systems makes a different claim about the balance between *freedom* and *equality* as this affects the relationship between the population of a country and their government as well as between individuals and groups. Liberalism emphasizes the greatest possible freedom for each individual person to exercise her or his own value preferences and consequently the minimum necessary action by government to secure the social order to make this possible. By contrast, socialism places greatest emphasis on equality between people as this can be seen both in opportunity and in outcomes, so government may legitimately restrict the freedom of individuals who enjoy advantages that are not of their own making in order that the opportunity of others is not impaired. Thus these two political systems tend to produce very different types of society.

A separation of politics from ethics is a relatively recent phenomenon. From the ancient thinkers such as Confucius (551–479 BCE) and Plato (429–347 BCE), through the late medieval and early modern period in the work of Thomas Aquinas (1224–1275 CE), Thomas Hobbes (1588–1679 CE) and John Locke (1632–1704 CE) and into the classic modern period of Immanuel Kant (1724–1804 CE) and John Stuart Mill (1806–1873 CE), these questions were not placed in separate categories. However, by the late twentieth century, politics and ethics often came to be been considered as different. In particular, some contributions to the field of professional ethics tend to discuss questions of individual morality while leaving matters of how the surrounding society is structured as a separate question. So, from this point of view, when the people professions make statements about particular values that have political implications they may be regarded as involving themselves in questions for which they have no particular competence. For example, should professional publicly criticize government policy if they consider it is harming the education, health, spirituality or social well-being of the population, or more especially of disadvantaged sections of the population?

Yet the people professions do make such statements, for example, in relation to *human rights* and *social justice* (IFSW/IASSW, 2004; ICN, 2006; WFOT, 2006; WMA, 2006). These two principles can be seen as uneasy partners, as one emphasizes the freedoms of individuals and the other the pursuit of equal opportunity and outcomes. Taken together they suggest a balance between sufficient freedom for people to live the life that they value while ensuring that no one is advantaged at the unfair expense of another. The extent to which statements supporting these values occur across the people professions can be taken as an indication that these professions regard such social conditions as *beneficial* to the pursuit of the goals of education and personal development, health, social well-being and so on. At the same time, in keeping with these values, individual members of the professions hold competing views about these balances. What tends to be agreed is that at the extremes of any political idea there are positions that are incompatible with the goals of the people professions, such as completely ignoring equality in order to achieve individual liberty or the suppression of individual liberty in order to achieve equality. Within these extremes, however, engagement with politics is a necessary element of professional ethics.

KEY TEXTS
- Clifford, D. and Burke, B. (2009) *Anti-Oppressive Ethics and Values in Social Work* (Basingstoke: Palgrave Macmillan), Chapter 6
- Daly, L.K. (2012) 'Slaves Immersed in a Liberal Ideology', *Nursing Philosophy*, 13 (1): pp. 69–77
- Emmerich, N. (2011) 'Whatever Happened to Medical Politics?' *Journal of Medical Ethics*, 37 (10): pp. 631–636
- Hughes Tuohey, C. (2012) 'Reform and the Politics of Hybridization in Mature Health Care States', *Journal of Health Politics, Policy and Law*, 37 (4): pp. 611–632

postmodern ethics

SEE ALSO **discourse ethics; pluralism; responsibility**

Modern thought can be understood as the era of science, in which systematic empirical inquiry has provided increasingly effective ways of understanding the world and acting on it. This can be seen in agriculture through the controlled breeding of animals and plants that provide great yields of food as well as in industry with the dominance of the production of iron and steel succeeded by electronics. In this period, the same approach has also been applied to society, with increasing rationalization in military systems, economics, government and health and social welfare. Indeed, in some respects, the material and social aspects of modernity are not separable.

In the second half of the twentieth century (CE), some philosophers started to challenge the dominance of this ways of thinking, especially as it applies to fields such as sociology, psychology, economics and politics. This approach argues that the use of all encompassing theories, which they call 'meta-narratives', is not sufficient to grasp the complexities of the world and most of all of people and societies. Because it follows modernism, this approach is called postmodernism. It lacks a more distinctive name because it is fluid, a collection of arguments against modernism rather than being a single position.

Postmodern ethics is critical of the modernist approach in the ideas of both *deontology* and *utilitarianism* because they apply the same way of thinking to everyone. Thus postmodern ethics rejects the *universalism* of a scientific approach to moral questions. A major figure in postmodern ethics is Zygmunt Bauman (b. 1925 CE) who wrote a major analysis of this idea (Bauman, 1993). The central idea here is that without compelling meta-narratives it is impossible to specify overarching ethical positions. Indeed, in his early statements on this, Bauman comes close to suggesting that formalized ethics are oppressive. Later he made other comments addressed specifically to people professions that appear to be more *pluralist* in that they make assertions about *human rights* and *justice* and the importance of pursuing such values, even though they do not always fit together very easily and they are highly contested (Bauman, 2001).

In summary, in as much as there is a single position on postmodern ethics, it is that if the plausibility of meta-narratives is questioned, then it is up to each person to make the best sense that they can of moral *responsibility*. In fact, such responsibility is the only value that can be addressed. However, this does not mean that people can simply pick and choose whether to feel responsible or simply to pursue their own benefit. Rather it is the opposite: in the absence of a meta-narrative, moral responsibility becomes all-encompassing because each person affects the lives of each other person with whom they are in any type of relationship. The moral web that this creates cannot be legislated, but it cannot be ignored. If I am to take my moral responsibility seriously (the same question that concerned Confucius, Plato, Kant and Mill), then I have to actively engage with the fluidity and uncertainty, working to make sense of such responsibility in all aspects of my life. Thus postmodern ethics is clearly neither 'anything goes' nor 'whatever' but even more demanding and challenging than the universal systems of either deontology or utilitarianism. For professionals this means having to constantly work out what is the 'good' and the 'right' action in each particular situation rather than being able to rely on ethical rules.

KEY TEXTS

- Gadow, S. (1999) 'Relational Narrative: The Postmodern Turn in Nursing Ethics', *Scholarly Inquiry for Nursing Practice*, 13 (1): pp. 57–70
- Gray, M. (2010) 'Postmodern Ethics' in M. Gray and S.A. Webb (eds), *Ethics and Value Perspectives in Social Work* (Basingstoke: Palgrave Macmillan)
- Hess, J.D. (2003) 'Gadow's Relational Narrative: An Elaboration', *Nursing Philosophy*, 4 (2): pp. 137–148
- Hugman, R. (2003) 'Professional Values and Ethics in Social Work: Reconsidering Postmodernism?' *British Journal of Social Work*, 33 (8): pp. 1025–1041

power (includes empowerment)

SEE ALSO **human rights; liberalism; oppression; politics; responsibility**

In the context of the people professions, the notion of power refers to the capacity of a person, a group of people or a social institution to make decisions and take action, in circumstances where there is a potential for conflict or resistance, whether such opposition actually occurs (Hugman, 1991). Thus, power can be seen in situations where an individual, group or institution sets an agenda that others accept as much as in circumstances where one side forces the other to accept. Indeed, it could even be said that power is greater when the authority or capacity of the one setting the agenda is accepted than when it is actively resisted. In professional relationships, this authority or capacity derives from the knowledge, skills and social position of practitioners. Service users, as well as employing institutions and the state, largely recognize such authority: it is why people seek the assistance of the people professions. We consult a medical practitioner, seek the help of a nurse, expect our children to be educated by people who are appropriately trained as teachers and so on, because we think that they have the capacity to provide this assistance.

It is this potential to affect the lives of service users, often (although not always) willingly, that presents the central ethical challenge to the people professions. This understanding of power is the reason moral *responsibility*, expressed both as personal commitment and in conforming to a *code of ethics*, is widely regarded as one of the most important features of professionalism. Furthermore, power is also exercised within and between professions, raising further ethical challenges. Therefore, power has to be seen as multi-dimensional, and following from this so do the ethical issues that arise from it.

Although an explicit concern with questions of power tends to be found in those professions that draw more heavily on sociological knowledge and theories, such as community development, social work and youth work (Clifford and Burke, 2009; Sercombe, 2010; Tesoriero, 2010), all the people professions are concerned with the issues to which this concept refers. Questions of *autonomy*, consent and *paternalism* all relate to the socially structured capacity of practitioners to exercise power over service users. From sociological ideas, some professions also pay great attention to other socially structured questions, such as the effects of sex and gender, 'race' and ethnicity, age, sexuality, disability and socio-economic class on the power of professionals.

From this, power has come to be seen as an ethical as well as a technical matter (Clifford and Burke, 2009). Seeking to ensure that service users can exercise autonomy, for example, is not simply a matter of following prescribed actions. It is also the way in which the ethics of the professions are played out in practice. The concept of 'empowerment' has become highly influential for this reason, with both ethical and technical implications. However, it is important to be clear about two problems with this notion. First, in the context of these professions it does not simply mean 'making people cope for themselves by withdrawing assistance'. It is for this reason that emphasizing the promotion of autonomy is key to understanding the idea. Second, empowerment is not something that is done 'to' or 'for' another person. What is both possible and desirable is that practices aim to promote the capacity of people (as individuals, families or communities) to exercise power for themselves: this is empowered autonomy. So while practitioners cannot empower service users by 'giving them power', how practice is undertaken can create the conditions in which service users may become empowered, both by helping service users to develop the necessary capacities and by not practising in ways that deny service users' moral autonomy.

Hugman (1991) argues that unless the people professions address questions of power and the social dimensions of relationships between service users and practitioners, fulfilling other aspects of professional ethics becomes very much more difficult if not actually impossible. Otherwise, practice may become oppressive through the failure to use power appropriately. Inequalities of power cannot be avoided in professional relationships, so ethical practice requires practitioners to make choices about how they use their power. Indeed, it raises the question of whether they do. Yet in making claims to various *principles* and *virtues* such as the promotion of autonomy, *beneficence, human rights, non-maleficence, respect* for persons and *social justice* the ethics of the people professions effectively commit their members to right action towards service users. In conditions of inequality that contribute to and even cause human needs, this cannot be achieved unless the relationship between power and inequality is consciously addressed. Thus, this suggests that in order to live up to their ethical statements, the people professions must attend to questions of power and the related issues of inequality and empowerment.

KEY TEXTS
- Adams, R. (2008) *Empowerment, Participation and Social Work* (Basingstoke: Palgrave Macmillan)
- Davidhizar, R. (2005) 'Benevolent Power', *Journal of Practical Nursing*, 55 (4): pp. 5–9

- Hugman, R. (1991) *Power in Caring Professions* (Basingstoke: Palgrave Macmillan)
- Starc, A. (2009) 'Nursing Professionalism in Slovenia: Knowledge, Power and Ethics', *Nursing Science Quarterly*, 22 (4): pp. 371–374

principles (including 'principlism')

SEE ALSO autonomy; beneficence; justice; non-maleficence; pluralism

A principle is a foundational truth or way of understanding the world that informs the way in which ideas are formed and applied. An ethical principle is the one that establishes a way of thinking about a moral issue. Many of the ideas that are presented in this book are principles that are used in the ethical deliberations of the people professions. Using principles to think about ethics means that they have to be applied and related to the specifics of a given situation, they are not simply rules that must be followed. In turn, this suggests that making principles the cornerstone of a profession's ethics requires practitioners to look consciously at the moral dimensions of their work.

A major impact of the explicit use of principles to construct ethics is represented by the approach that has come to be known as 'principlism' (Beauchamp and Childress, 2009). This approach specifies the various principles that together form the foundation of ethics. Beauchamp and Childress address biomedical ethics, which can also be understood broadly as health ethics, and identify four principles that they argue form the basic structure of such ideas: *autonomy, beneficence, non-maleficence* and *justice*. Originally proposed in the 1970s (CE), this approach has become the dominant perspective in the biomedical and health professions, as well as influencing other such as social work (Banks, 2012) and youth work (Sercombe, 2010). While the possibility that these ideas can be understood as if they were simple rules or slogans has been questioned (e.g. Gallagher, 1999, among others, refers to it as the 'Georgetown mantra'), the growing body of work discussing the way in which principlism can inform deep debate shows that this is not necessarily the case and that it offers a sophisticated approach to the range of issues that must be considered when thinking about all ethical aspects of a professional situation.

An important part of Beauchamp and Childress' (2009) argument is that the four principles do not necessarily simply fit together as if they were pieces of a jigsaw puzzle. To bring them together requires conscious deliberation. There are times when applying one principle can lead to a violation of another. For this reason, practitioners must learn to 'weigh and balance' the principles with each other (Beauchamp and Childress, 2009, pp. 14–25). They go on to say that this is the process that most people go through in ordinary life situations. The principles that they assert for the people professions are identified from such an observation. Because they say that these ideas are shared widely throughout many societies, they call it 'common morality'. Banks (2012) also specifically develops this notion in relation to social work, where she identifies the balance to be found between *deontology, utilitarianism, virtues* and *social justice* to be the key question.

This is clearly a type of *pluralist* ethics, as their description is very similar to that of Hinman (2012) and other pluralist moral philosophers. Hinman takes a slightly different approach in that he adds principles such as understanding, tolerance, standing up against *evil* and fallibility. While these are different to the four biomedical principles, they can be set alongside to add to the range of ideas available to practitioners. Pluralism provides the philosophical basis on which it is possible to address ethics as an element of practice to be engaged with and developed continually throughout one's career and not simply as a rule book. Broadly, the balance sought in Hinman's ideas can be summarized as knowing when and how to act and being comfortable with acting differently in different circumstances without seeing this necessarily as arbitrary or inconsistent. Understanding and tolerance concern the capacity and willingness to listen to others' points of view and to consider them (without implying that they have to be accepted), standing up against evil suggests knowing how to see when something is simply 'different' and when it is 'wrong' and fallibility involves a sufficient degree of humility to be able to question oneself and listen to criticism from others. A clear example of this can be found in the concern with research ethics in the people professions, often centred on the idea of informed *consent,* which seeks to avoid the evils of past research practices in which subjects have been treated in inhumane ways, sometimes even to the excess of torture and death. Conscious rejection of such practices draws on all four of the principles outlined by Beauchamp and Childress (2009), in that it seeks to promote autonomy and justice while practising beneficence and non-maleficence.

The integration of principles that form the modern consensus in the health professions can assist in creating the possibility of openness and dialogue that are necessary for other *values* to be achieved within and between the professions themselves as well as with service users and the wider society.

KEY TEXTS

- Banks, S. (2012) *Ethics and Values in Social Work*. 4th edn (Basingstoke: Palgrave Macmillan), Chapter 2
- Beauchamp, T.L. and Childress, J.F. (2009) *Principles of Biomedical Ethics*. 6th edn (New York: Oxford University Press)
- Gallagher (1999) 'The Ethics of Compassion', *Ostomy/Wound Management*, 45 (6): pp. 14–16
- Karlsen, J.R. and Solbakk, J.H. (2011) 'A Waste of Time: The Problem of Common Morality in *Principles of Biomedical Ethics*', *Journal of Medical Ethics*, 37 (1): pp. 588–591

r

relativism (cultural, ethical)

SEE ALSO pluralism; subjectivism; universalism

Ethics is the 'conscious reflection on our moral beliefs' (Hinman, 2012, p. 5). This means that it concerns deliberations about the values that each person holds about the way in which a good human life should be achieved. Yet the differences between people, communities and whole societies mean that the wider our consideration the more it is likely that difference and disagreement will be found. One solution is to define key values as necessary for all people to live a good life – this position is called *universalism*. Against this, others argue that ethics must be understood in each particular context. This position is called relativism, as it is based on the claim that values and hence ethics are relative to each situation. At its most individualistic level, relativism can lead to *subjectivism*, in which each person's subjective view of the world is regarded as discrete and equally plausible (Rachels, 2010). On this basis, there is no basis for choosing between values other than they happen to be the preferences of the person holding them. However, the major positions in relativism do not go this far, but see some commonalities between people based either on shared culture or on agreement about key ethical ideas.

The first of these significant forms of relativism is that of cultural relativism. This position holds that insofar as values differ between cultures there is no basis on which they can be compared, other than to note their empirical differences. However, within each culture, there is an expectation of shared values. Thus, for example, while it is possible to speak about common norms among people from European cultural backgrounds, or to recognize *African* values or Asian ethics as distinct, each is regarded as distinct and able to be evaluated only from its own relative stance. Thus, cultural relativism argues that each set of norms or values must be treated as integral in itself. On this basis, it is not possible to make evaluative comparisons between them. So, the notion of *filial piety* is reasonable within an Asian cultural context but could not be applied in making ethical judgements about people from European backgrounds, for instance. Indeed, one of the major differences between modern European and other cultural norms might be said to be that of an individualistic as against a collectivistic view of the moral status of human persons. From this, relativism argues that what is good from an Asian perspective may or may not be good in any other culture, and so on. For members of the people professions, this means that arguments about certain practices as harmful to education, health or social well-being must be questioned as assertions of particular cultural perspectives. Female genital cutting and marriage and childbirth involving girls still in puberty are examples of cultural practices where members of the professions may be challenged about the imposition of European (or 'Western') values when they argue that these practices are harmful. Similarly, the concern demonstrated across these professions for *human rights* (IFSW/IASSW, 2004; ICN, 2006; WFOT, 2006; WMO, 2006) may be criticized as being an inappropriate promotion of a particular cultural perspective.

Ethical relativism is different. When people hold divergent values but are members of the same culture or community, this can be understood as relativism with regard to the principles that are used to explain and act on these values. To take Asian values and norms as an example, while some people may argue that a focus on human rights is inappropriate (effectively a 'Western imposition'), others may argue for human rights in an Asian context. Similarly, not everyone in European, African or other cultural settings uniformly accepts the value of human rights. Under these circumstances, each person must form their own position and beyond that there is no particular standard or point of reference by which any one position can be evaluated in relation to any other. It is this form of relativism that can blur into subjectivism, which is, as Hinman puts it (2012, p. 34), 'often conveyed through a shrug of the shoulders and a "whatever"'.

From a professional practice perspective, there are several problems with relativism. First, in relation to culture, what exactly defines a discrete culture? Especially in multi-cultural contexts, the boundaries between cultures are not fixed and impermeable. Ideas are exchanged and people find ways of living alongside one another.

Beyond that, people can rethink their values when exposed to alternative points of view. Cultures do not remain unchanged over time, but develop as old ideas are adapted or new ideas accepted. Third, it is never clear precisely whose understanding of a culture should prevail. Different members of a culture may hold divergent interpretations of norms and values. So if a practitioner is working with someone from another culture, it might be most appropriate to ask individuals how they see their cultures. In many situations, this would be a helpful way to proceed, as it would relate actions to the values of the person most directly affected. However, then we are left with the question of value differences between any one individual's understanding of their culture and the ethics of a particular profession and of the practitioner. Relativism offers no particular way of addressing how these competing value claims can be reconciled or a decision made between them. Some accommodations are made, such as in the scope for a medical practitioner or a nurse who objects morally to abortion not to work in such services, or to refer to someone who is seeking an abortion, but there are also many situations where such solutions are not available. In comparison, the practice of female genital cutting provides a different type of challenge for practitioners in countries where it is illegal, as it cannot be so easily regarded as 'simply a matter of how things are done in this culture.' A further example, if less immediately contested, is that social workers, teachers and youth workers may all find themselves working with diverse groups in which some general or shared norms have to prevail for a group to function, which sets a limit on the extent to which each young person's values can be accepted within the group.

For these reasons, although relativism may appear attractive from a standpoint that is seeking to be open, oppose *oppression* and to value *equality*, in practice it may be very hard to achieve completely as it does not lend itself easily to forming a clear position that can be shared across a community that is defined by membership of a distinct profession as compared to a culture or another type of community.

KEY TEXTS
- Häyry, M. (2005) 'A Defense of Ethical Relativism', *Cambridge Quarterly of Healthcare Ethics*, 14 (1): pp. 7–12

- Hugman, R. (2013) *Culture, Values and Ethics in Social Work* (London: Routledge), Chapter 5
- Hyun, I. (2008) 'Clinical Cultural Competence and the Threat of Ethical Relativism', *Cambridge Quarterly of Healthcare Ethics*, 17 (2): pp. 154–163
- Rachels, J. (2010) *The Elements of Moral Philosophy*. 6th edn (ed, S. Rachels) (New York: McGraw-Hill), Chapter 2

religion and spirituality

SEE ALSO existential ethics; Indigenous ethics; ma'at

Many modern ethical concepts have their origins in religious beliefs. This is evident in all parts of the world. Religious and spiritual ideas address what it is to be human, the way in which human beings relate to the natural world, questions of how people should behave towards one another and so on. In that sense, they are concerned with morality.

Religions differ in terms of the way in which they understand the idea of the divine: is this a transcendent being or a power or force; is this a singular entity or a plurality and do the claims of a particular religion apply only to members of a faith or to all people? Indeed, the claim that there is no such thing as spirituality (atheism) could even be described as a position on religion. Consequently, except in the most mono-cultural context, there are likely to be differences between people about these things that will affect their views about moral questions. Not only will professional practitioners encounter service users with different beliefs to themselves but they will also be working with colleagues who hold diverse beliefs. Given the strong influence of religion on ethics, this means that there are likely to be differences of values between people in all of the work of the people professions.

As the social influence of religion has weakened, in Western cultures in particular, Hinman (2012) identifies three possible constructions of the relationship between religion and ethics based on human reason: religion always has precedence; religion and reason should be compatible; and reason always has precedence. It is this, he suggests, that actually forms the basis of disagreement about religion in societies where more than one approach to this matter is recognized. Because modern forms of the people professions are based on reason, there is a tendency for religion and spirituality not to be regarded as appropriate as a basis for *codes of ethics*. Where these identify religion at all, it is in relation to a requirement for practitioners to be *respectful* to service users regarding their particular beliefs, which in any case are often defined as cultural rather than religious as such.

Yet there are sometimes problems in practitioners being able to accept and acknowledge service users belief systems within their work, where these conflict with the demands of practice. One widely canvassed example of this is the religious prohibition on the receipt of blood in medical treatments by members of particular faiths (Tschudin, 2003; Beauchamp and Childress, 2009). For some practitioners, this may be resolved by reference to notions of *autonomy*, *dignity* and so on where the person is making such a decision for her or himself but will be resisted when the decision is being made for someone else who lacks the capacity to express a decision (such as a child). Other such examples include different views about abortion, end-of-life decisions, out of home care of children (such as fostering and adoption), decisions concerning the involvement of children in various activities in schools and more generally in relation to professional interventions in families such as in relation to family violence and relationship problems.

Another major ethical issue for the people professions is that in countries where religion and spirituality have come to be regarded as private matters, through the impact of modernization and the rise of reason as the dominant way of seeing the world, these questions may not always be addressed by practitioners in responding to service users' needs. Yet when this is an important aspect of a service user's life, not to attend to this can mean that important aspects of the person's needs may not be adequately addressed. This in turn raises questions about tolerance and acceptance of difference and the extent to which practitioners are able to work with service users (and colleagues) who have divergent values while still maintaining their own beliefs.

A further ethical issue is raised by the extent to which educational, health, social welfare and youth services are provided by religious or faith-based organizations. Where this occurs, the extent of which differs between countries, there can be problems of inclusivity and exclusivity (Clifford and Burke, 2009). Should such organizations only provide services for their own faith communities, should they receive public funds to do so and should they be able to make moral judgments about who they will provide services to? Clifford and Burke (2009) see a connection between these questions and issue of culture and ethnicity in particular. However for them religion also raises challenges of *equality*, especially regarding gender and sexuality, as the positions of women and of lesbian and gay people are often regarded differently by traditional religious perspectives compared to men and to heterosexuals, thus not fitting easily with professional values based on *human rights* and *social justice*.

KEY TEXTS

- Holloway, M. (2007) 'Spiritual Need and the Core Business of Social Work', *British Journal of Social Work*, 37 (2): pp. 265–280
- Hugman, R. (2013) *Culture, Values and Ethics in Social Work* (London: Routledge), Chapter 7
- Medrum, H. (2011) 'Spirituality in Medical Practice: How Humanitarian Physicians Draw Their Boundaries with Patients', *Integrative Medicine: A Clinician's Journal*, 10 (3): pp. 26–30
- Reimer-Kirkham, S. (2009) 'Live Religion: Implications for Nursing Ethics', *Nursing Ethics*, 16 (4): pp. 406–417

respect

SEE ALSO **deontology; dignity; human rights; values**

This idea functions as both a *principle* and a *value*, informing ethics in all the people professions. In many ways, it can be seen as one of the most important moral concepts as it informs or supports other dimensions of ethics, such as *autonomy, compassion, dignity* and *rights*. Respect is the recognition of the humanity of each person, as having the capacity to take moral *responsibility* of their choices and preferences. It asserts that every person is to be regarded as a moral actor, a subject and not an object.

The most significant modern understanding of respect as a core element in ethics comes from the philosophy of Immanuel Kant (1724–1804 CE). Kant argued that the defining aspect of humanity is rationality and from this he developed a rational system of ideas in which what is right and wrong can be demonstrated by logical argument (*deontology*). Underpinning this approach is the notion of the 'categorical imperative'. This is an idea that has to be followed because it is logically correct. The categorical imperative that Kant proposed is: 'Act only on that maxim through which you can at the same time will that it should become a universal law' (1991, p. 84). To this he added what he called a practical imperative: 'Act in such a way that you always treat humanity, whether in your own person or the person of any other, never simply as a means but at the same time as an end' (Kant, 1991, p. 91). The first of these is a claim that it is illogical not to apply the same moral principle to everyone's actions. The second concerns the illogicality of regarding some people as objects and not as subjects, when in doing so one is acting as a subject; this in turn fails to conform to the requirements of the first version of the imperative because it effectively says 'I can treat you as an object when I expect to be regarded as a subject.' In that case, the claim behind the action (the maxim) is not being applied to everyone equally.

The most common example that is widely discussed, because Kant himself used it (1991, pp. 67–68), is that of the choice between telling the *truth* and lying. Social relationships depend on *trust*, in that if we cannot rely on each other's statements, the fabric of everyday life would quickly break down. If it is necessary to have to check constantly if another person did, is doing or intends to do what she or he says, then normal relationships would be impossible.

Kant relied on an argument based on rationality to explain why respect for the humanity of all people is the basis for ethics. However, while this is important from some other perspectives, it can be seen as inadequate to explain everything about respect as a core principle and value. For example, I respect my family, my neighbours and my colleagues not simply because of a duty to rationality, but also because of my social and emotional relationships with them. Respect is also connected to the *care* that people might express towards one another, for example. It can also be a part of attention to questions of *social justice* in the way in which a person who recognizes that they have particular *power* and authority in a situation pays attention to respect for the humanity of the people whose lives they affect through their actions.

In practice situations, service users often have to be treated in ways that they would not normally. This can include telling someone they do not know very well intimate details about their lives, relationships, feelings and bodies, exposing themselves metaphorically and at times literally to people in order to receive assistance in resolving a problem or meeting need. In such situations, respect is made real through the practitioner's actions. This includes listening carefully to what service users say, enabling dignity to be maintained and keeping details about a person private to the greatest extent possible.

Some forms of *paternalism*, such as withholding facts about a situation from a service user, do not fit easily with respect. Where the practitioner has clear evidence that a service user does not want to know everything, it may be plausible that this can be *beneficent* towards the person. However, as discussed in a separate section in this book, when a decision is made to act in this way it should be a deliberate and conscious choice made for a specific purpose and not simply a practice routine. Under such circumstances if respect is to be maintained towards the service user, then the principle of paternalism should be regarded as an exception. Similarly, overriding a service user's wishes in making decisions should be done only for reasons that can be justified by reference to the prevention of a greater harm. Protecting the life of another person is one such example, which can be encountered in situations involving questions of child maltreatment or certain actions arising from mental health problems. Teachers face a different challenge in this respect, in that they may more often be called on to act in ways other than that for which an individual student may wish. Respect is shown by being able to explain clearly to the student so that she or he may learn about the reason for actions; it involves responding to the student as having the capacity for moral reasoning that is appropriate to their age and development (Carr, 2000).

Although the development of the idea of respect in modern professional codes of ethics tends to rely on a Kantian approach, it can also be found in other ethical systems as well. *African*, Asian and *Indigenous* ethics all place respect at the centre of their thinking. Exactly how respect is demonstrated can differ between cultures, but the underlying principle and value are the same: to accord full humanity to each person. Browne (1995) describes practice as a nurse of European cultural background working with an Inuit community in Canada, in which respect was a primary value in establishing a good relationship with patients. This involved, amongst other things, allowing women to maintain modesty while being physically examined, taking time to explain procedures and actions and listening to patients' descriptions of their problems. So although some aspects were culturally different between the service users and the practitioner, the basic value was clearly understood and shared by both. This example also points to one of the reasons respect may sometimes be breached: it often needs to be deliberate. Busy practitioners working with limited resources can at times either forget to or be prevented from demonstrating respect in their actions.

KEY TEXTS

- Banks, S. (2012) *Ethics and Values in Social Work*. 4th edn (Basingstoke: Palgrave Macmillan), Chapter 2
- Browne, A.J. (1995) 'The Meaning of Respect: A First Nations' Perspective', *Canadian Journal of Nursing Research*, 27 (4): pp. 95–110
- Geisinger, J. (2012) 'Respect in Education', *Journal of Philosophy of Education*, 46 (1): pp. 110–112
- Kunyk, D. and Austin, W. (2012) 'Nursing under the Influence: A Relational Ethics Perspective', *Nursing Ethics*, 19 (3): pp. 380–389

responsibility

SEE ALSO care (duty of, ethics of); codes of ethics; consequentialism; wisdom

The *principle* of responsibility provides a way of understanding the connection between notions such as *autonomy* and *rights*, as well as between the capacity to act and the *consequences* of actions. It emphasizes that these other principles and factors have to be seen as part of human relationships. While I may reasonably claim that I have the capacity to make my own moral judgements and that I have certain expectations that social structures and the actions of others will not impede me from acting on them, at the same time I also have to acknowledge that other people also make the same claims and have the same expectations. So I must also consider how my choices and actions will affect other people. The same morality that gives me autonomy and rights places obligations on me to have a regard for the way in which my actions are actually interactions that have consequences for others. Thus, I can be called to give an account of why I have made certain choices, unless my actions genuinely affect no one but myself. However given the social nature of humanity, it is hard to think of a world in which a person's actions have no potential implications whatsoever for anyone else in any way.

One of the ways in which the principle of responsibility is considered is as the other side of rights. Insofar as rights language refers to people as the holders of rights, for these to be achieved it is usually necessary for others to act in ways that either do not impede or actually facilitate the achievement of the right. The others in this relationship are considered to be the bearers of responsibilities in the sense of having the obligations to uphold the person's rights.

The *ethics of care* approaches the idea of responsibility differently. Tronto (1993) argues that awareness of the impact that one has on others creates a series of moral choices for action. Rather than understanding responsibility as obligation, the ethics of care proposes that it is consciously embraced as part of any relationship that a person seeks to nurture and sustain. Thus responsibility requires action, as it becomes the way in which one person attends to another person. This involves being mindful of, listening to, seeking to understand and choosing how to act towards the other.

Both the rights based and the ethics of care approaches to responsibility share the implication that the morality of social relationships makes each person accountable to others. Accountability in this sense means that others can expect to be able to ask the person to explain choices and actions. It is about 'giving an account' of why these things were chosen or done as opposed to some alternate possible things. In some circumstances, accountability can imply that the other(s) to whom the account is given can exercise authority over the person. The idea of 'responsibility to an employer' is an example of this. However, in many situations, responsibility is moral rather than legal or procedural. Even then, however, there may be an expectation that the person gives an account in the sense of being able to explain and justify why she or he has acted in a particular way. The idea of 'responsibility to service users' is an example of this in many practice contexts. Clearly, where service users are the direct employers of professionals, the two senses merge into one interaction.

In complex societies responsibilities to different people may be in competition or even conflict with each other. Banks (2012,

p. 165) distinguishes between services users, one's own profession, an employing agency and the wider society as the main 'others' to whom responsibilities may be held. To this can be added that the responsibilities felt towards one's family or neighbours may be different from those held towards 'society' in a more general and diffuse sense. For example, should a practitioner place responsibilities towards a service user ahead of those towards her or his spouse and children? It is actually very difficult to be prescriptive about this and Banks, among others, argues that in everyday practice people make varying decisions based on balances between the seriousness of the circumstances towards which they feel responsibility. This may lead to responsibility in one area taking precedence when on another occasion a different decision is reached. It seems unreasonable to interpret an ethic of *service* such that responsibilities to service users always over-ride everything else, but at the same time reasons for placing one's family, colleagues or self ahead of service users must be defensible in terms of seriousness, likely consequences and so on. So, for example, a person whose life or safety is at risk or who faces great distress might take precedence in most circumstances, while needs that are less immediate may be balanced against promises made to family or a colleague.

Finally, recent arguments about *postmodern ethics*, which emphasizes that all matters of morality are indeterminate (i.e. they cannot be specified in advance by formal rules but must be worked out in concrete situations), suggest that responsibility is to be found in *courage* to accept that other people may not agree with choices that are made. The willingness and capacity to provide an account of one's reasons for making a particular choice are highlighted in this understanding. It is not always possible to say which of a range of alternate choices is the best; indeed, there may be good reasons for choosing more than one, or for not positively preferring any. Under such circumstances, *wisdom* consists of knowing what others may think (which in the context of professional life includes a *code of ethics*), making the best judgement that one can and then being prepared to accept the obligation to resolve consequences that follow from it, including facing the moral opinion of service users, peers and others.

Many of the texts that practitioners and students in the people professions consult about ethics do not discuss responsibility in detail, or even explicitly in some cases. Yet this is a notion that lies behind a concern with ethics. Professionals exercise *power* in relation to service users and the wider society, through knowledge, skills and the positions that they occupy. Without an explicit connection to the idea that the exercise of such power calls for responsibility on the part of practitioners, the very idea of professionalism by itself can become a 'conspiracy against the laity' as Shaw (1911) so critically put it.

KEY TEXTS

- Banks, S. (2012) *Ethics and Values in Social Work*. 4th edn (Basingstoke: Palgrave Macmillan), Chapter 6
- Clancy, A. and Svensson, T. (2007) '"Faced" with Responsibility: Levinasian Ethics and the Challenge of Responsibility in Norwegian Public Health Nursing', *Nursing Philosophy*, 8 (3): pp. 158–166
- Nortvedt, P., *et al.* (2011) 'The Ethics of Care: Role Obligation and Moderate Partiality in Health Care', *Nursing Ethics*, 18 (2): pp. 192–200
- Stefkovitch, J. and O'Brien, M.G. (2004) 'Best Interests of the Student: An Ethical Model', *Journal of Educational Administration*, 42 (2): pp. 197–214

S

service

SEE ALSO codes of ethics; responsibility

In a discussion of youth work ethics, Sercombe (2010, p. 10) asserts that '[w]e do not provide a service we serve.' Service is not simply the tangible acts that practitioners provide for service users but rather it should be understood as a moral commitment to act well in the provision of skills and knowledge to meet needs and to pursue the valued goals of the profession with service users. In the case of youth work, this is the social and personal development of young people. Koehn (1994) extends this idea to all professions, arguing that their moral purpose is to pursue the values that are congruent with their nature, whether this is education, health, *justice*, social well-being or a combination of these.

Underlying the idea of service is the ethic of commitment. For many members of the people professions, this is the commitment to service users, primarily, and only to the skills and knowledge that provide a vehicle for service as a secondary matter. While it is necessary to be skilful and knowledgeable, this is not to be valued by itself but for the purpose of being able to serve others. Banks (2006, p. 83) refers to the oath of the South African Black Social Workers Association, which begins with the words 'I swear', making a promise to service users of a commitment to serve. There are clear parallels here with the Hippocratic oath of the medical profession (Beauchamp and Childress, 2009, p. 149). This is a rather different approach to formal *codes of ethics*, in that the idea of commitment to service implies the practitioner incorporates ethics into her or his professional self, whereas it is possible to regard codes as external, for example seeing them as rules or guidelines.

Commitment to service as a primary ethic demands that the practitioner places the interests of the service user ahead of her or his professional interests. A particular action may be more interesting, provide an opportunity to learn or instruct others, be more financially profitable or simply more convenient, but if this is not the best action in terms of the service user's interests, then the ethic of service argues that it should not be undertaken. Service is other-directedness.

A possible problem with using a commitment to serve as the basis for professional ethics is that there are many people who have the needs with which the people professions work. Unless this commitment is tempered with the reasonable claim that the practitioner has to look after her or himself and to attend to other relationships such as family, there is a risk that professionalism begins to appear as a type of self-sacrifice. This seems to be requiring too much. Practitioners need to maintain their own health and relationships to be in a position to be able to serve others. In that respect, the ethic of service contributes to a balanced approach rather than being an overarching value. As with *responsibility*, commitment to service lies at the heart of ethical professionalism and is one of the moral factors that make professional ethics distinctive.

KEY TEXTS

- Helm, C.M. (2006) 'Teacher Dispositions as Predictors of Good Teaching', *Clearing House: A Journal of Educational Strategies*, 79 (3): pp. 117–118
- Sercombe, H. (2010) *Youth Work Ethics* (London: Sage Publications), Chapter 2
- Tschudin, V. (2003) *Ethics in Nursing: The Caring Relationship.* 3rd edn (Oxford: Butterworth-Heinemann), Chapter 1
- Walz, T. and Ritchie, H. (2000) 'Gandhian Principles in Social Work Practice: Ethics Revisited', *Social Work*, 45 (3): pp. 213–222

social justice

SEE ALSO **equality; fairness; justice; oppression; utilitarianism**

Although the *principle* of *justice* is widely discussed as one of the common moral values, professional ethics also talks specifically about *social* justice (Banks, 2006; Beauchamp and Childress, 2009). Since the time of Confucius (551–479 BCE) and Plato (429–347 BCE), philosophers have tended to regard the achievement of a just society to be closely related to the existence of just individuals. However, this can often be understood as emphasizing the actions of individuals as the origin of justice. Recognizing the social dimension of justice focuses attention on the way in which social structures and relationships can be just or unjust.

The focus of concerns about social justice tends to be towards groups or classes of people rather than individuals. For example, a lack of *equality* in opportunity and outcome according to sex, 'race' and ethnicity, (dis)ability, age or sexuality are all ways in which societies can be seen to be unjust. The underlying moral claim is that when such differences arise from factors that are not an essential aspect of a situation, then an *unfairness* is perpetrated. This goes further than simply arguing that a more equal distribution of opportunity and outcome might be better, as it asserts that injustice denies people the potential to live a truly human life; in that sense, it denies their humanity. In addition, identifying such matters as social justice makes it clear that inequalities of this kind arise because of social structures and relationships independently of the actions of any one individual.

Discussions of these questions within professional ethics tend to be more explicit in those professions that draw on social theory as part of their knowledge base. Community work, social work and youth work particularly emphasize this concept, seeing it as foundational to ethics, and some discussion can also found among nurses and teachers (Carr, 2000; Tschudin, 2003; Butcher *et al.*, 2007; Sercombe, 2010; Tesoriero, 2010; Banks, 2012). Many of the problems and issues that they address are now understood as at least partly, if not entirely, caused and affected by inequalities in social structures and relationships.

However, while discussions in medicine tend to examine 'justice' without the prefix 'social', in reality they are often asking the same sorts of critical questions. In Beauchamp and Childress' (2009, ch. 7) analysis of justice, they focus on similar concerns as those found in other texts, including unequal distributions of access, opportunity and outcome in health care that arise from social factors, as well as the causation of ill-health. Community medicine and public health are areas of the profession that are directly concerned with these matters, but all aspects of medicine, they argue, should take them into account.

Young (1990) has argued that the important question in matters of social justice is not the distribution of resources but oppression. In other words, what matters most is not that one person might get some more resources than another but that this occurs on the basis of the advantages enjoyed by some people (such as men, ethnic majorities, people who do not have disabilities, younger and middle-aged adults and heterosexuals) at the expense of others. So if a practitioner is concerned to promote social justice, when considering to whom scare resources should be allocated she or he may think it legitimate to favour people who are disadvantaged. For example, a young single mother who lives in social housing and whose income consists of social security payments is a person who ought, on this basis, to receive particular attention. More widely, it should be of concern to practitioners, policy makers and managers that members of ethnic minorities are statistically more likely than other groups to have poor health outcomes and access to health care while at the same time being over-represented in the criminal justice system. This can be seen with Aboriginal people in countries such as Australia, Canada, New Zealand and the United States; it also applies to non-Indigenous groups, such as Black communities across Europe and North America. On the basis of social justice, such figures point to the way in which disadvantage is socially structured and is not simply the result of bad individual life choices.

Some critics have argued that the identification of a social dimension to questions of justice is not acceptable because it has the effect of leading to attempts to create different social structures, which in turn limits the *freedom* of individuals to hold differing values (Nozick, 1974). Against this, Rawls (1972) has developed what is probably the most influential view in the people professions, which locates questions of justice within social structures and relationships. In brief, Rawls argues that the opportunities that we have in life are at least partly a matter of chance, in whether we are born male or female, in a particular ethnic group, with particular abilities or disabilities and so on. Thus, a just society is the one in which such factors do not create such unfairness that people are denied the opportunity to live a decent life. At the same time, as a *liberal*, Rawls leaves room for some differences of opportunity and outcome, but only where these are not dependent on unfair advantage. Achieving such a society is seen as impossible by many critics, either from the liberal individualist side (such as Nozick), because it still limits the personal freedoms of some people for the good of all and so has a *utilitarian* element, while for radical egalitarians it fails because it allows for the continuation of some inequalities.

The concern of professions about social justice is expressed in some ethics documents, including *codes of ethics* and other such statements (IFSW/IASSW, 2004; ICN, 2006; WMA, 2006). While these documents make some reference to the difficulties of agreeing between people as to exactly what sort of relationships and actions constitute social justice, they are in agreement that a balance must be struck between redressing inequalities and disadvantages that come from social circumstances and valuing difference and diversity, including the opportunity for people to exercise their abilities and to benefit when they do so. For this reason, the people professions should be seen as having a legitimate role in *political* debates and decisions about structures, policies and practices that cause or otherwise impact on the needs and issues that they address.

KEY TEXTS

- Banks, S. (2012) *Ethics and Values in Social Work*. 4th edn (Basingstoke: Palgrave Macmillan), Chapter 2
- Beauchamp, T.L. and Childress, J.F. (2009) *Principles of Biomedical Ethics*. 6th edn (New York: Oxford University Press), Chapter 7
- Crigger, N.J. (2008) 'Towards a Viable and Just Global Ethics of Nursing', *Nursing Ethics*, 15 (1): pp. 17–27
- Johnstone, M. (2011) 'Nursing and Justice as a Basic Human Need', *Nursing Philosophy*, 12 (1): pp. 34–44
- Reisch, M. (2002) 'Defining Social Justice in a Socially Unjust World', *Families in Society: The Journal of Contemporary Social Services*, 83 (4): pp. 343–354

subjectivism

SEE ALSO **emotion; postmodern ethics; relativism**

Subjectivism can be considered as a particular form of *relativism*. It describes a perspective from which all moral questions are addressed by reference to the personal preferences of each individual. That is, the basis of morality is each person's own subjective view of the world. This presents particular difficulties for the people professions because each of them in some way seeks to make changes in the world for the benefit of others. In deciding what should be the focus of professional attention, a sufficient amount of agreement must be reached on what is wrong, why it is wrong and what should be done to change it. Of course, this could be seen as possible simply through a collection of a great many individuals who all just happen to agree with each other. However, even if this provides a majority point of view, it is still just a matter of what people personally prefer: there is no moral content. Consequently, ethics is collapsed into 'etiquette' or 'aesthetics'. As many philosophers have pointed out deriving an 'ought' (such as 'I think this should happen') from an 'is' (such as 'this is what I see the majority of people are preferring') is not a legitimate argument (a view originally advanced by David Hume [1711–1776 CE]). Something else is required, which is a standard of moral evaluation that is external to the preferences of individuals in this sense.

If taken to its logical conclusion, the subjectivist perspective not only does not allow for any shared moral understanding to be developed but also leads to a situation where such questions will tend to be resolved through the use of social power. To take the example of the ill-treatment of children, with which many of the people professions are actively concerned, that this is seen as undesirable does not rest on the personal views of professionals, but has been extensively debated socially and the policies and practices that are now in place in many countries reflect wide agreement about the morality of caring for children (Houston, 2001). Arguments for and against this can be examined for the assumptions they contain, as well as their logic and implications. In this way, the morality of child welfare is not simply a matter of personal preference. Even when people defend physical chastisement, they do so on the grounds of culture (such as 'it is regarded as appropriate to do that here') or effectiveness (such as 'other means of discipline mean that children do not learn right and wrong') both of which have a normative content to which such justifications are appealing. In other words, such defences of physical chastisement are based on shared moral norms and values, not on subjectivity (as in 'I just happen to think it's ok').

Banks (2012) makes the point that in a profession matters of ethics have to be shared to have meaning. Although each practitioner has their own values, in being part of a distinct occupation there are some limitations on the way in which subjectivity can be used to justify actions that are clearly contrary to the shared views of the broader profession (e.g. as expressed in a *code of ethics*). If the individual practitioner's values are in conflict with those of the wider occupational community, then choices have to be made about continuing to practice as a member of the relevant profession or in a particular context.

KEY TEXTS

- Houston, S. (2001) 'Transcending the Fissure in Risk Theory: Critical Realism and Child Welfare', *Child and Family Social Work*, 6 (3): pp. 219–228
- Hugman, R. (2005) *New Approaches in Ethics for the Caring Professions* (Basingstoke: Palgrave Macmillan), Chapter 7
- Leget, C. and Olthuis, G. (2007) 'Compassion as a Basis for Ethics in Medical Education', *Journal of Medical Ethics*, 33 (10): pp. 617–620

supererogatory (action)

SEE ALSO **beneficence; benevolence; service**

Commonly shared moral values, such as the ethics of a profession, establish norms of good practice. These bring together elements of duty and *virtue* to create ideals. However, in some (perhaps many) instances, people 'go beyond what is required' and act in ways that can be seen as 'selfless', 'generous' or even 'heroic'. These acts are called supererogatory.

Beauchamp and Childress (2009, p. 48) state that four criteria have to be met in order for an act to be supererogatory.

(1) It has to be optional and possible, that is neither demanded nor excluded by normal standards.
(2) It has to exceed which is expected by normal standards as good.
(3) It has to be done deliberately for the benefit of others: it is beneficent and not done for self-interest.

(4) It has to be good in and of itself and not simply something that is done with good intentions.

There are many areas of practice in the people professions where there is an understood limit to the demands that can be expected of anyone, for example because of risks or other potential costs. Caring for people with highly infectious or contagious diseases is one such instance. So is working with people who have severe challenging behaviours or where the work routinely brings the practitioner into contact with human waste. Ironically, many of these roles are relatively low status within the professions and/or attract lower remuneration than ordinary practice.

One of the areas in which supererogatory action can be seen is in practice undertaken in humanitarian and aid contexts. These may require people to take a degree of risk, such as in situations of natural disasters or of human conflict, and as a consequence supererogatory action cannot simply be demanded of anyone in order for them to be regarded as a good member of the profession. It is both optional and, where there are costs and risks, it is beyond the normal level of what is praiseworthy. It is also clearly undertaken for the benefit of others and is good by itself, in that it provides interventions for people in vulnerable situations who otherwise do not have sources of help. However, not all developmental work comes into this category, as some is done on normal levels of remuneration and in safe conditions. So, even though such work may be beneficent and good by itself, it does not meet the criteria of supererogatory action.

The work of people professions can appear supererogatory to those for whom the content and focus of such practices are seen as challenging, whether emotionally, morally, psychologically or even (in some instances) financially. However, from the perspective of these professions themselves, supererogation lies in those choices and actions that are 'above and beyond' by the standards of the professions and not by wider views.

KEY TEXTS
- Beauchamp, T.L. and Childress, J.F. (2009) *Principles of Biomedical Ethics*. 6th edn (New York: Oxford University Press), Chapter 2

- Carlisle, D. (2010) 'Beyond the Call of Duty: Physiotherapists Do Not Have to Be at the Top of Organisations to Effect Considerable Improvements in Patient Care', *Frontline*, 16 (11): pp. 20–22
- Dickinson, S.M.D. (1995) 'Beyond the Call of Duty: Memoirs of a Nurse in Hiroshima ... Excepts From Misako's Writings from 1979', *Journal of Practical Nursing*, 45 (2): pp. 23–26

sustainability

SEE ALSO care (ethics of); futility; responsibility; utilitarianism

In recent years recognition of the moral implications of the impact of human action on the natural world has increasingly become part of ethical debate. In what has become a pivotal analysis, Singer (1975) set out a *utilitarian* argument that non-human animals should be regarded as sentient beings and so be taken into account as such in making deliberations about the balance of well-being and misery arising from actions. For Singer, this means that using animals to meet the needs of humans is morally unacceptable if it causes pain or suffering. Thus, for example, he argues against eating meat.

This approach is taken further by Midgley (2001) who draws on the concept of 'Gaia' (an understanding of the world as a self-sustaining living organism) to argue that the individualism underpinning modern Western ethics is no longer plausible. In its place, Midgley argues, we should use notions of connectedness and relationship to consider moral questions. This not only means the connectedness between human, or between humans and animals (as suggested by Singer) but also between humans and the entire natural world, whether seen as animate or otherwise. So, all actions that have an impact on the natural world have an inherent moral dimension. In this argument, Midgley agrees with Singer that the capacity of humans for abstract reason, language and other faculties that earlier philosophers had suggested placed humans in a separate moral realm do not give humans superior moral claims (whether seen as needs or *rights*) but rather emphasizes the greater *responsibilities* held by humans. In other words, being human does not mean that our needs or rights should reduce or even deny the needs of other species or the inanimate world; it points to the way in which human capacities create moral obligations precisely because we are able to consider the impact of our actions.

Central to this approach is the idea of sustainability. If it is possible for human reason and language to provide the basis for moral consideration, this can include thinking about the way in which actions will change the balance of the natural world and its capacity to survive. In simple terms, humans can choose whether to use the material in such a world that it is able to be self-sustaining or at such a rate and in such quantity that it becomes depleted (in other words, it gets used up).

Gower (1992) summarizes the argument of environmentally aware ethics in asking the question 'what do we owe to future generations?' The answer is that while he does not consider the present generation should sacrifice everything for future generations, acceptance of this argument sets limits on how we might understand current well-being. However, if the material well-being of the current generation (in developed countries) has been gained at the expense of future generations, these have been morally bad choices.

Although this can be seen as type of utilitarian argument (focused on the balance of well-being and misery of different groups of people), it also includes elements of the *ethics of care* in that it is relational. This supposes that a generation can reasonably anticipate what might be the preferences of a future generation. To some extent, this can easily be answered by the fact that all animal life requires air, water and food – at the very least the present generation has a moral obligation to leave a world in which these necessities of life are available to others. Beyond that, however, is the suggestion of Gower, Midgley and others, that we only have to think two generations into the future in making choices and these are people that we are likely to know. This leads to the concept of the '200 year present': a person alive now, assuming a natural life-span of about 75 years, can have known two generations before (grandparents) and two generations into the future (grandchildren). (Indeed, this is the experience of the present author, having known great-grandparents who were born in the 1870s (CE) and a great-niece born in the early twenty-first century who, on average figures, may expect to live into the 2090s.) In this way, the ethics of sustainability is relational because 'the future' is not an abstract notion but has a human face and at the same time can be connected to the past.

The implication for the people professions is that all aspects of practice and policy should be considered in terms of sustainability. If this ethical challenge is addressed, the pursuit of ever more complex health and social care interventions and systems has to be examined in terms of the overall resource costs. For example, putting large amounts of funding into the extension of the human life-span is a conscious moral choice in a world in which many people do not survive to the average age because they die of diseases that already can be cured or prevented. This may have a particular meaning in care for older people, in which a human rights perspective points to equal access to treatment and care irrespective of a person's age, while a more utilitarian argument may set a limit on interventions for all people, for example, by considering that the amount of resource used to keep someone alive in pain and lacking *dignity* may be regarded as disproportionate. Where expensive interventions are *futile*, then this becomes a stronger criticism.

At a more systemic level, the idea of sustainability also raises questions about the type of service structures and policies that may be developed. The current generation of the people professions has to face the challenge of creating structures and policies that can be sustained, socially, economically and ethically into the future. One side of the argument suggests that this is simply a matter of being realistic in planning, so that too much is not attempted too quickly. Against this, however, is the view that the burden of proof about any development (whether of a drug, an intervention or a policy) lies with those who propose it and not with those who might question its appropriateness. This view of sustainability is that it is a change that must be justified and not the maintenance of current good practice.

KEY TEXTS

- Besthorn, F.H. (2002) 'Radical Environmentalism and the Ecological Self: Rethinking the Concept of Self-Identity for Social Work Practice', *Journal of Progressive Human Services*, 13 (1): pp. 53–72
- Dwyer, J. (2009) 'How to Connect Bioethics and Environmental Ethics: Health, Sustainability, and Justice', *Bioethics*, 23 (9): pp. 497–502
- Gower, B.S. (1992) 'What Do We Owe Future Generations?' in D.E. Cooper and J.A. Palmer (eds), *The Environment in Question: Ethics and Global Issues* (Buckingham: Open University Press)
- McKinnon, J. (2008) 'Exploring the Nexus between Social Work and the Environment', *Australian Social Work*, 61 (3): pp. 256–268

t

trust

SEE ALSO care (duty of); honesty; integrity; virtue

A relationship between a service user and a professional practitioner almost always requires the disclosure of information about the service user, whether this is about their body, their personal relationships or their social circumstances. Because the people professions, by definition, are concerned with those areas of life in which people cannot cope with their problems unaided (England, 1983, p. 13), such sharing of information is highly sensitive. Central to the way in which service users and practitioners approach each other is the idea of trust, which forms the moral basis of the relationship between the two.

Trust can be understood as the confidence that each side of the relationship is able to have in the other. For the service user, it is the expectation that in telling the practitioner things about oneself appropriate help will be received. Being a service user makes a person vulnerable physically, socially and emotionally. So having sufficient confidence in the practitioner is vital for the service user to be open and comfortable in receiving help. For the practitioner, it is the expectation that the service user will share what is necessary for appropriate help to be provided and will engage in what is needed in order for the assistance to be received.

The idea of trust in the professional relationship has a long history. The oath of Hippocrates (c. 460–370 BCE) for medical practitioners includes the promise not to hurt people who seek help. The idea of 'hurt' here is not so much about the temporary experience of unavoidable pain but rather refers to long-lasting damage that might be caused through lack of *competence* or an appropriate level of *care*. Practitioners are not always conscious of the considerable power that they have over the lives of service users. Being worthy of trust may not require such consciousness at all times, but it does demand that practitioners think and act on the basis that they can be called to account in this respect. So to be trustworthy implies that the practitioner will be honest, treat people with dignity, maintain confidentiality and privacy and display other aspects of regard for the moral integrity of the service user. In this sense, the idea of trust is related to *virtue* ethics because it concerns the character of the practitioner. The trustworthy practitioner is someone whose character shows traits on which service users can rely to have confidence that they will not be damaged by receiving help.

One example of trustworthiness in practice is in the way in which personal information is used. Because of the social implications of seeking help, for example, possible stigma or shame, it is important that service users can have confidence that practitioners will not disclose information outside the professional relationship. Breaches of *confidentiality* can easily destroy trust, although in complex service systems this is sometimes easily misunderstood (see the separate section in this book on this topic). Similarly, if practitioners make promises that they are then unable to keep this can reduce or destroy trust in the professional relationship; likewise, giving wrong information (or even actually lying) will make trust very difficult. Or, again, if the practitioner has to make a decision, or forms a view that the service user does not like this may damage trust, even though it can be considered necessary from the basis of professional theories and methods. So, maintaining trust requires that practitioners are very clear in communication with service users and with each other. This involves both listening carefully to service users' understandings and expectations as well as finding ways of ensuring that professional ideas and information have been understood. It means being careful with all aspects of the relationship.

Although it is also important that practitioners can trust service users (to give the right information, to be open and *honest* and so on) the responsibility for this can often rest with practitioners. Given the imbalance of power that is inherent in most professional relationships, there are many instances where service users will be trustworthy in this sense when they are able to trust practitioners. Examples of this include young people being open in their relationships with social workers, teachers and youth workers, or people with mental health problems responding openly to health professionals. This aspect of trust has parallels with the ethics of *care*, in which the caring relationship is fulfilled with the responsiveness of the cared-for person. This notion suggests that the ethics of a helping relationship is, therefore, not only the responsibility of the professional. Yet it is in the responsiveness of service users, in also being trustworthy, that practitioners can see the impact of their own trustworthiness.

KEY TEXTS
- Beauchamp, T.L. and Childress, J.F. (2009) *Principles of Biomedical Ethics.* 6th edn (New York: Oxford University Press), Chapters 2 and 8
- Dinç, L. and Gastmans, C. (2012) 'Trust and Trustworthiness in Nursing: An Argument-Based Literature Review', *Nursing Inquiry,* 19 (3): pp. 223–237
- Englund, T. (2011) 'The Potential of Education for Creating Mutual Trust: Schools as Sites for Deliberation', *Educational Philosophy and Theory,* 43 (3): pp. 236–248
- Sykes, R.L. (2004) 'Ethical Attributes and Professional Skills Development', *The New Social Worker,* 11 (2): pp. 4–5

truth

SEE ALSO **deontology; discourse ethics; fidelity; honesty; integrity; trust**

At face value, the idea of truth may appear obvious: a statement is either correct or it is not. However, Hugman (2005) summarizes the arguments of German philosophers Apel, Gadamer and Habermas that claims to truth vary according to the area of life that is being considered and the way that these are understood. This leads to the idea of three different 'types' of truth: propositional, normative and subjective (as listed in Table 5).

The difference between these forms of truth can be illustrated with the following example. The statement that 'all helping professionals must act as advocates for service users' cannot be regarded as propositionally true. This is not a claim that can be considered as a fact. In contrast, the statement 'the codes of ethics of nurses, social workers and youth workers say that they should seek to act as advocates for their service users' can be examined as propositional, as it can be tested by being compared to the texts of the relevant codes of ethics. At the same time, the original idea can be said to be

Type of truth	Meaning
propositional	a statement (about an object, an event and so on) directly communicates a *fact* about a aspect of the world
normative	a statement communicates something that conforms to what is regarded as *right* in relation to knowledge, values and expectations
subjective	a statement communicates the sense of a person's beliefs about her or his own subjective experience

TABLE 5 *Three types of truth*

true to the extent that large numbers of people in these professions hold the claim to be normatively right. It does not cease to be true in this sense even if some individual members of these professions subjectively hold a different view.

The important point here is that ethics is not a matter of fact: it is a question about norms and values. At the same time, it cannot adequately be reduced to what each individual person subjectively thinks. The statement 'I do not like the way in which my profession's ethics emphasizes advocating for the needs of service users' may be subjectively truthful, but that is a different matter.

Another problem that comes from the common understanding of truth as propositional facts is that it can be difficult to ensure that all aspects of a situation are stated. The tradition in Anglophone legal systems of declaring that a statement is 'the truth, the whole truth and nothing but the truth' comes from the way in which different interpretations can be put on a statement depending on whether some parts are missed out or additions are made. In both cases what is said is factual, but the meaning changes because of the context.

So, 'simply telling it like it is' cannot be seen as quite so simple. For practitioners, therefore, it is important to see truth, rightness and truthfulness as different aspects of 'truth'. To achieve this requires awareness that truth by itself not only enables the world to be grasped, so that the best interventions are used, for example. It is also part of *fidelity, honesty, integrity, trust* and so on. In other words, virtuous practitioners are those who are able to be clear about the claims to truth that they are making and to communicate this clarity to others, including service users. This is both in terms of their statements being true in some way (the common sense view of truth) and of their capacity to distinguish between propositional facts, normative rightness and subjectivity.

For Banks (2006, pp. 55–56), the notion of 'truthfulness' is better used to describe the practitioner who seeks to develop this degree of clarity in their thinking, speech and actions so that others are then able to trust. Beauchamp and Childress (2009, pp. 288–295) extend this argument by looking at the reasons that practitioners might be untruthful for apparently good reasons. In situations of giving bad news, such as of a medical diagnosis that a physician has reason to think the patient will misunderstand, can be regarded as a form of *paternalism*. This might be considered *beneficent*. However, they go on to argue that truth-telling is a strong value that should only be limited when another stronger principle commands attention. In this regard, they also differentiate between 'partial disclosure' that can be added to later and deliberate lying in the sense of making statements that are propositionally, normatively and/or subjectively false. However, they make very clear that they only condone this position when there is a genuine intent and practical plan to make the correct information available as soon as is seen as possible. Yet they continue to hold reservations about departures from the view that truth-telling should be the moral default position. In other words, the burden of justification rests with those who argue against seeking to tell the truth and not those who think that finding ways of telling the truth is normatively right.

KEY TEXTS

- Begley, A.M. (2008) 'Truth-Telling, Honesty and Compassion: A Virtue-Based Exploration of a Dilemma in Practice', *International Journal of Nursing Practice*, 14 (5): pp. 336–341
- Hugman, R. (2005) *New Approaches in Ethics for the Caring Professions* (Basingstoke: Palgrave Macmillan), Chapter 8
- Richard, C., Lajeunesse, Y. and Lussier, M. (2010) 'Therapeutic Privilege: Between the Ethics of Lying and the Practice of Truth', *Journal of Medical Ethics*, 36 (6): pp. 353–357
- Walz, T. and Ritchie, H. (2000) 'Gandhian Principles in Social Work Practice: Ethics Revisited', *Social Work*, 45 (3): pp. 213–222

u

ubuntu

SEE ALSO community; Indigenous ethics; ma'at; responsibility; social justice; virtue

This *African* concept has many translations. However, they all share common elements that are encapsulated in Tutu's (1999) explanation that it concerns the interconnectedness of people. A widely used rendition of this concept in English is 'I am because we are; and since we are, therefore I am' (Mbiti, 1990, p. 160). From this perspective, it is not possible to be a person in isolation from others: to be human is to have a shared rather than an individual social and moral identity.

While the word 'ubuntu' itself is from the Xhosa language of South Africa, the concept has equivalents in all of the sub-Saharan languages. From this Graham (2002) argues that it is necessary to see Africa as having a shared value system much as it is possible, for example, to talk about European or Asian values. Ubuntu shares this with the principle of *ma'at*. As with ma'at, ubuntu emphasizes the communality of human life. Thus, it is very different from the individualism that has come to define European ethics since the medieval period. From such a foundation, the moral framework of African thought has to be approached quite differently.

Ubuntu can be considered as a *virtue*. Certainly, Tutu addresses it in these terms, arguing that a person has (or does not have) this quality, which is shown when the person:

> is open and available to others, affirming of others, does not feel threatened that others are able and good, based from a proper self-assurance that comes from knowing that he or she belongs in a greater whole and is diminished when others are humiliated or diminished, when others are tortured or oppressed.
>
> (Tutu, 1999, p. 31)

Furthermore, as with the European view of virtues, these characteristics cannot be seen simply as ideas that someone holds, but are qualities that must be seen in the way that a person acts, especially in relationships with others. The person with ubuntu displays this in all aspects of her or his life. Ubuntu is also based on notions of moral identity and obligation rather than of *rights*. It speaks of what a person ought to be and to do towards others; only by implication does it make a claim that others should act in the same way.

From this, it can be seen that African values may be incompatible with modern ethics that is derived from the European Enlightenment, precisely because the latter is individualistic. The same difference can be seen between Western perspectives and *Indigenous* ethics. So, a major problem for professional ethics can be encountered in situations where the service users' world-view is based on ubuntu. For example, from the perspective of ubuntu concepts such as self-determination and confidentiality are regarded very differently to the individualistic understanding that informs modernistic professional practice. Where this is the case, service users may expect members of their families or their wider communities to be involved in considerations of problems, making plans and then in implementing them in ways that might be regarded as inappropriate from other cultural perspectives. This can be seen in the saying 'it takes a village to raise a child,' which carries the implication that the well-being of each young person is not simply the responsibility of particular parents but is shared with the wider family and with neighbours.

The professional practitioner who has and displays ubuntu is a person who is committed to the *service* of others. Her or his practice is focused primarily on the needs and well-being of the service user rather than on a technical interest in the nature of the problem. It embodies a view of professionalism as service rather than as a virtuoso performance of esoteric skills or as social status. It is not that skill is unimportant: the incompetent practitioner can help no one and may cause harm. However, within the communally oriented world-view, skills and knowledge find moral significance in their use to assist others, as against the way in which they create an identity for the practitioner.

While ubuntu may appear incompatible with a Western, individualistic view of rights, it resonates more with the concept of *social justice.* Relationships that are guided by ubuntu promote acceptance, reciprocity and the sense of moral equality. This provides a point of connection between African, Indigenous and Western values, alongside the idea of virtues or moral qualities. Indeed, by linking concerns with social justice and equality with virtues, ubuntu emphasizes that the actions of each person can contribute to a just society. This is illustrated by the custom in some parts of Southern Africa when a criticism is made of a group or community and an argument is presented for ways in which a situation might be improved, a speaker concludes with the statement 'starting first with myself'. In this way, group membership is emphasized over individual identity and the person takes responsibility for the group's response to problems and issues. This is the origin of Gandhi's (1869–1948 CE) statement that we should seek to 'be the change that [we] want to see in the world', which was influenced by the time he spent as a lawyer in South Africa (Majmudar, 2005).

For the people professions, this means that the promotion of good practice originates with each practitioner who seeks to understand and to act on moral values such as ubuntu as the basis of their professionalism. From this point of view, professional ethics does not start or finish with a formal *code of ethics* but rather with a concern to seek good practice for oneself in relationship with others. It also implies that a practitioner with ubuntu will be concerned with the overall practice of a team in which they might work and to support good actions on the part of others and not simply with her or his own achievements.

KEY TEXTS

- Malaudzi, F.M. *et al.* (2009) 'Suggestions for Creating a Welcoming Nursing Community: Ubuntu, Cultural Diplomacy and Mentoring', *International Journal for Human Caring*, 13 (2): pp. 45–51
- Mbiti, J.S. (1990) *African Religions and Philosophy*. 2nd edn (Oxford: Heinemann Educational Publishers)
- Mji, G. *et al.* (2011) 'An African Way of Networking around Disability', *Disability & Society*, 26 (3): pp. 365–368
- Ross, E. (2008) 'The Intersection of Cultural Practices and Ethics in a Rights Based Society: The Implications for South African Social Workers', *International Social Work*, 51 (3): pp. 384–395

- Waghid, Y. and Smeyers, P. (2012) 'Reconsidering "Ubuntu": On the Educational Potential of a Particular Ethic of Care', *Educational Philosophy and Theory*, 44 (Supplement 2): pp. 6–20

universalism

SEE ALSO codes of ethics; deontology; pluralism; relativism; utilitarianism

Should the same moral values apply to all people? Should a practitioner treat all people in the same way in ethical terms? The position of universalism holds that they should. In this sense, it is the opposite of *relativism* (which is the view that values are relative to the context, especially with regard to culture). Debates about universalism tend to concentrate on two possible aspects: whether morality derives from a common human nature; and whether it is possible or necessary to claim that one particular way of thinking about ethics is paramount or overarching.

The first element of universalism is that of a common human nature. This position holds that there is an underlying commonality to the moral nature of humanity that means all people should always be treated with the same regard. An example of this is Kantian *deontology*, which argues that the distinctive feature of being human is to have a rational capacity for moral awareness and responsibility. Deontology then asserts that, following logically from this, because humans are moral creatures then each and every person is owed the highest regard by all others. In this way, ethics has a universal foundation, because morality is shared by all humanity.

Utilitarianism similarly includes all people equally, in its argument that the preferences of each person should be given equal weight in making a moral calculation about the best outcome of choices and actions. It is universal in that it states no person's ideas or values should be seen as greater or lesser than anyone else's.

An important criticism of universalism is that although it seeks to treat people equally, it does so in a way that tends to deny the important differences that can be found between the lives that people value in various contexts. The result is that only some particular views of what is good are accepted. This can then lead to a position where the values of only some groups are taken as the standard by which 'common humanity' is defined.

One approach that has sought to deal with this criticism is that of Amartya Sen and Martha Nussbaum in their development of the concept of 'human capabilities' (e.g., see Sen, 1983; Nussbaum, 2000). Nussbaum identifies common aspects of the way in which societies are organized that provide people with the possibility of pursuing the life that they value. Such capabilities include the opportunity to think for oneself, to experience emotions and the physical senses, to make choices within the finite nature of the world and to form relationships. Without being able to achieve these things, Nussbaum argues, life is not fully human because the shared aspects of humanity require these things. At the same time, the actual choices that are made, for example, valuing a particular type of family and other relationships, will be different according to culture and other factors.

The other criticism of universalism is that it leads to claims that one approach to ethics is paramount or overarching. Kekes (1993) calls this perspective 'monism' (only *one* way of understanding values). This leads, ultimately, to the claim not only that the lives of all people ought to be evaluated in terms of the same moral ideas but also that there is one best way of understanding what those moral ideas might be. An example of this in modern ethics is the continuing debate through the twentieth century (CE) between deontology and utilitarianism, with the proponents of each point of view asserting the superiority of their favoured approach.

Against this, *pluralism* argues that it is possible to acknowledge that both the values that people hold and the concepts and ideas used to understand and discuss them can reasonably be different between people without having to accept a totally relativistic conclusion. In doing so, it continues to give the same moral status to all people and so while it rejects a monistic view that there is only one right answer to the question 'how should we live?' in remains universal in that same stock of values is understood to be shared by people in very different situations, such as the importance of life, *honesty*, commitment to one's own family and community, *respect* for others and so on. Nagel (1979), for example, calls this 'common morality'.

For professional practitioners, such a debate may appear to be quite removed from day today life. *Codes of ethics* provide a common set of moral standards that are taken to apply to the whole of a profession – in that sense they are universal. The implication is that all service users should expect to be regarded and treated ethically in the same way. Yet such values and the practices that follow from them are not fixed, either between social and cultural groups or over time within the same society. For example, Beauchamp and Childress (2009, p. 207) give the example of the way in which acceptance of *paternalism* as morally acceptable in medical care has now given way to increased attention to patients' *rights*. At the same time, they also note that in other circumstances health professionals may act differently towards people from ethnic minority groups than they might towards those from the mainstream culture, precisely as a way of maintaining the same broad underlying values of *respecting* each person for who she or he is. In this sense, the general intention is universal while the means by which it is achieved is different.

Central to the claims made opposing discrimination and *oppression* against people on the basis of sex, ethnicity, religion, physical and mental abilities and disabilities, age and sexuality is the notion that human rights and social justice are universal values. Without this understanding, arguments, for example, that older people should receive the same quality of care and service as younger people, or that ethnic and 'racial' minorities should be valued as highly as service users who are in the ethnic and 'racial' mainstream, are severely weakened. For this reason, universalism plays an important part in contemporary professional ethics, as it provides the basis for human rights and social justice to be seen as important. The problem is to hold these values while at the same time recognizing that the way in which they are implemented may need to vary according to the identity and situation of each service user. For this reason, professional ethics cannot be reduced to sets of rules or left to others to decide; it concerns all members of each profession.

KEY TEXTS

- Englund, T. (2011) 'The Potential of Education for Creating Mutual Trust: Schools as Sites for Deliberation', *Educational Philosophy and Theory*, 43 (3): pp. 236–248
- Healy, L.M. (2007) 'Universalism and Cultural Relativism in Social Work Ethics', *International Social Work*, 50 (1): pp. 11–26
- Hugman, R. (2013) *Culture, Values and Ethics in Social Work* (London: Routledge), Chapter 4

- Schwarz, S.H. (2007) 'Universalism Values and the Inclusiveness of Our Moral Universe', *Journal of Cross-Cultural Psychology*, 38 (6): pp. 71–28
- Tangwa, G.B. (2004) 'Between Universalism and Relativism: A Conceptual Exploration of the Problems in Formulating and Applying International Biomedical Ethics', *Journal of Medical Ethics*, 30 (1): pp. 63–67

utilitarianism (includes act, ideal, preference and rule utilitarianism)

SEE ALSO consequentialism; justice; principles; social justice

In many ways, this is one of the most influential approaches from moral and political philosophy that affects ethics in the people professions. It is the most widely known form of *consequential* ethics. The ideas underpinning utilitarianism were originally set out by an English philosopher, Bentham (1748–1832 CE), who argued that right action was concerned with the maximization of pleasure and the minimization of pain. In response to criticisms that this was too crude a way of understanding human actions, J.S. Mill (1806–1873 CE) restated it in terms of happiness (by which he meant what would now be called 'well-being') and misery. In both formulations, and those that have followed, utility is regarded as the goal to be achieved through the balance of outcomes for all people who are involved in or affected by a particular act. Thus, for example, if many people benefit from the act and only one person is adversely affected, then it may be a good choice. However, as Hinman (2012, p. 13) points out, appropriate measures of utility are actually very difficult to quantify. For example, it is possible to interpret this notion in such a way that it would be acceptable to harm one person deliberately in order to benefit one thousand. Taken to the extreme, this appears to allow that murdering a homeless young person with no hope for a good life to harvest organs to save the lives of many other people would be 'good'. Yet this is precisely the type of crude understanding that Mill was concerned to reject. He refined the idea by setting limits that scaled the cost to any one person, so that such harm cannot be acceptable no matter how many others might benefit. In the twentieth century (CE), further attempts were made to refine this approach, notably 'ideal' utilitarianism (the achievement of *justice, freedom* and other ideals) and 'preference' utilitarianism (the balance of whether people are able to pursue personal preferences). Modern utilitarians base their arguments on such principles, such as Singer's (2002) advocacy for a concern with *social justice*.

Two particular mechanisms for achieving the balance of utility have also been suggested. These are act utilitarianism and rule utilitarianism (Freeman, 2000). The first of these states that those acts that produce the greatest utility should be performed. The problem with this approach is that it assumes the person acting can accurately predict the consequences. A more subtle way of thinking about how to achieve the best outcome is to consider the rule that if followed ought to produce utility. In this way those who are making judgements do not need to be concerned about their ability to be accurate in this respect.

One of the ways in which utilitarian *principles* have been highly influential in the people professions is in the practice of 'triage'. This concept derives from the Great War of 1914–1918 (CE), where faced with large numbers of casualties medical and nursing personnel had to choose whom to treat first and, by implication, who might then die while waiting for assistance. So wounded soldiers were divided into three groups (hence 'tri-age'): those who were very likely to live and who did not require intensive help; those who were very likely to die anyway and where pain relief was all that could be offered and those who might live but required an urgent response to do so. On this basis, the last category was given priority for medical attention. This is an example of rule utilitarianism, in that although the actual consequences for any one individual could not be predicted with total accuracy, the basis of such decisions ought to produce the best balance of well-being against (potentially avoidable) misery.

This practice is found today in the emergency or casualty rooms of hospitals, especially in developed countries that have public health services. While it may be normative under other circumstances for people to be seen by treating professionals in order of their arrival or of an appointment, in such circumstances judgements must be made about who is in the greatest need of immediate attention. Thus, the person with a more minor problem may have to wait a long time, while the person who has a life-threatening but treatable condition will be seen immediately. In addition, in non-life-threatening situations, the same principle is often applied to decisions about the allocation of practitioners' time and the use of resources: which young person should the teacher or youth worker give their time to now and which service user with serious problems should the remedial therapist or social worker see this afternoon? As neither time nor resources are limitless, such decisions are part of the everyday work of practitioners.

The *universal* approach that is implied here, that people are treated equally according to the objective facts of their need, may be equitable when matters of life and death are being considered, but a great deal of professional practice does not involve such decisions. In other settings, such as non-urgent health care, schools and colleges, human services agencies, youth centres and so on, resources are also limited and in many of these social factors that have a material or structural element may need to be taken into account. For example, should the single mother living in public housing receive a priority response from a social worker over someone whose circumstances are materially better but whose emotional distress appears to be greater? Does it (indeed, should it) make any difference if either of these service users is a member of an ethnic minority community?

Reconciling the idea of preference, utilitarianism with practice in many aspects of the people professions is very difficult. In circumstances where the service user is not able to state their own value preferences, or where practitioners have a responsibility to act independent of the preferences that are stated (statutory child protection and mental health emergencies are examples of this), decisions have to be made on some other basis. Insofar as utilitarianism informs such choices rule utilitarianism is often the principle that is applied. Research by Osmo and Landau (2006) with social work students showed that in the classroom deontological principles were favoured, while in practice settings the same students reported making decisions based on rule utilitarianism. (The present author has observed the same difference between the statements of students across the health professions and practice in multi-disciplinary health settings.) It appears that when faced with the difficult task of trying to find ways of making decisions about scarce resources (including their own time), practitioners have to reach 'on balance' judgements. At the same time, they often still hold to values that are supported by other principles, which in combination with the decisions that they have to make effectively produces an 'ideal utilitarian' element alongside the more clearly identifiable 'rule utilitarian' model that this research identifies. In this way, the realities of practice rarely demonstrate any of the types of utilitarianism in their 'pure' form but as contributing aspects of a *pluralistic* ethical position. This suggests that educators should consider promoting a deeper understanding of utilitarianism, especially among students and beginning practitioners.

KEY TEXTS

- Beauchamp, T.L. and Childress, J.F. (2009) *Principles of Biomedical Ethics*. 6th edn (New York: Oxford University Press), Chapter 9
- Clifford, D. and Burke, B. (2009) *Anti-Oppressive Ethics and Values in Social Work* (Basingstoke: Palgrave Macmillan), Chapter 4
- Freeman, S.J. (2000) *Ethics: An Introduction to Philosophy and Practice* (Belmont CA: Wadsworth), Chapter 5
- Rachels, J. (2010) *The Elements of Moral Philosophy*. 6th edn (New York: McGraw-Hill), Chapters 7 and 8

V

values

SEE ALSO codes of ethics; principles; virtues

Banks (2012, p. 8) points out that the term 'values' is widely used but can have many different meanings. Yet, as ethics is the way in which we consciously think about values (Hinman, 2012, p. 5), it is important that we understand what values are and the role that they play in thought and action. For most moral philosophers and applied ethicists values are regarded as those things in life that people consider worth pursuing. In this sense, values are the goals of our lives, those things that are regarded highly and are believed to be important enough to spend time and effort trying to achieve. Values are the descriptions given to those things that comprise a good life. Values are the judgments that are made when people evaluate the world.

Kekes (1993, p. 44) makes an important point that values can be moral and non-moral. An important part of the distinction between the two is that non-moral values can occur naturally, whereas all moral values are the product of human thought and action. An example of a non-moral value is 'health', which is something that people regard very highly and which has both natural and socially created dimensions. Health is something that people devote their resources and efforts to achieving. Having health is then seen as a measure of a good life. In contrast, an example of a moral value is 'honesty'. This is entirely a social concept and cannot be said to have a natural aspect. As a facet of people's characters and actions, honesty may also be seen as important in the achievement of a good life, but here it is on the basis of the way in which it creates the conditions of particular sorts of human relationships and behaviours.

The values of the people professions can be seen as both moral and non-moral. Koehn (1994) presents an argument that, more than anything else, professionalism should be regarded as the pursuit of non-moral values: education, health and (social) well-being. It is these goals to which the people professions should be directed, as opposed (say) to the social status of practitioners, salary levels or the intrinsic interest to be found in esoteric knowledge and skills. In short, these non-moral values are the reasons why the people professions exist.

Moral values in these professions can be seen as the ways in which professional objectives are accomplished. However, this does not mean that they are simply means to other ends; they are also ends that should be pursued in themselves. It is, rather, that in achieving education, health or social well-being there are good ways of doing so. Without the achievement of moral values, non-moral values (goals) are diminished and may actually not succeed. As other sections of this book explain, moral values can be examined from three perspectives: duties (such as in *deontology*), *consequences* (such as in *utilitarianism*) and intrinsic character (as in *virtue* ethics). However, each of these only offers a framework for thinking about ethics (technically called 'meta-ethics'). In other words, they are a means to achieving the ends of more specific values. It is these more specific statements of value that are normative – in other words, indicate what counts as good. Examples include: *care, fairness, justice, respect, responsibility, rights* and *truth*. These are all statements of the qualities found in human actions and relationships, which people regard as important because they make life more 'fully human'.

Banks (2012, p. 7) also draws attention to the difference between professional values and personal values. It is possible that the shared values of the profession as a whole will not include all the values of each individual member. For example, the value statements of professions do not normally include commitment to particular religious or political ideologies (at least in the sense of formal religions or political parties). It may even be that there are conflicts of values between professions and some of their individual members. A commonly used example of this in ethical discussions is in relation to abortion. This is a practice that no profession would now regard as inherently 'wrong', yet there may be individual practitioners who consider it to be so. For some this conflict is resolved by choosing to work in roles removed from the value conflict (so, e.g., some allied health professionals, nurses or social workers may choose to work in other areas of health services); however, for others such as some general medical practitioners, it may not be possible to draw such a clear line and this may be resolved either by subordinating personal values to those of the wider profession or by making clear to patients that for such a service they should look elsewhere.

Codes of ethics are the formal statements of each profession concerning their values. In practice, there is a high level of agreement between them (see, e.g., Hugman, 2005, pp. 143–144). They also tend to be congruent with the wider values of the societies in which they are located, although this cannot be taken for granted. Indeed, there are examples where the values of the people professions stand as a criticism of some societies, such as in the statements by national and international professional associations condemning inhumane treatment of prisoners, the state sanctioned use of torture and other violations of human rights (IFSW/IASSW, 2004; ICN, 2006; WFOT, 2006; WMA, 2006). In this way values, both moral and non-moral, form the 'identity' of each profession, which in Koehn's (1994) terms makes them 'professions' as opposed to simply being highly technical occupations.

KEY TEXTS
- Gabel, S. (2011) 'Ethics and Values in Clinical Practice: Whom Do They Help?' *Mayo Clinic Proceedings*, 86 (5): pp. 421–424
- Koehn, D. (1994) *The Ground of Professional Ethics* (London: Routledge)
- Nagel, T. (1979) *Mortal Questions* (Cambridge: Cambridge University Press), Chapter 9
- Rathburn, G. and Turner, N. (2012) 'Authenticity in Academic Development: The Myth of Neutrality', *International Journal for Academic Development*, 17 (3): pp. 231–242

virtue

SEE ALSO **phronesis; values; wisdom**

A person may be described as virtuous if she or he displays particular characteristics. The good allied health professional, doctor, nurse, social worker, teacher or youth worker is one who performs that function well. More than this, good practitioners are those who perform their functions well because they have developed the capacity to be the right kind of people for the role. In this sense, virtue ethics is the ethics of character.

Historically, the notion of virtue as the basis for ethics derives from ancient Greece, especially the thought of Aristotle (384–322 BCE). The good human life, in this way of looking at ethics, is one in which people flourish in the sense of being able to live truly human lives. Virtue ethics teaches that this occurs when the characters of individuals enable the society as a whole to flourish. The well-being of individuals and of the society are seen as interwoven. (The Greek terms *eudaimonia* that means flourishing has the implication of 'doing well'; sometimes it can also be translated as 'happiness', which in modern English has a somewhat different implication; see MacIntyre, 1998.) So the virtuous practitioner is not only the one who demonstrates good qualities in her or himself, but in doing so contributes to the well-being of others and of their society. Yet virtue lies not in outcomes or in performing moral duty but in the qualities that lead to flourishing.

A further aspect of Aristotle's thought that helps in thinking about virtues is that he saw them as a mid-point between excess and deficiency of characteristics (Hinman, 2012, p. 259). In this way, a virtue sits between two qualities that can be considered as vices. An example of this might be in the quality of *compassion*, which is widely regarded as good in a member of the people professions. However, it is possible to have too much compassion, which would be called pity, as well as too little that results in a callous disregard for the plight of others. Pity here can be understood as a feeling towards the plight of others that seeks to assist but does so on the basis of condescension, belittling the capacities of the other and so taking over that person's moral responsibility: in effect it is as dehumanizing as is callousness. This can be seen in a situation where the practitioner rushes to do things for people when it would be more helpful for the person to do the task for themselves, even if with support, either because this promotes their sense of dignity or because they gain in their own competence.

The exact list of virtues discussed by Aristotle reflects the society in which he lived. Not all of those qualities would now be considered as relevant. So to identify the virtues of the people professions, it is necessary to look at their functions. These can be described as assisting people to achieve education, health and social well-being (as discussed elsewhere in this book, e.g., under the theme of *values*). In order to do this, good practitioners need to display particular qualities, which might include: *altruism, benevolence, care, compassion, competence, courage, fairness, harmony, honesty, integrity, justice, loyalty, respect* (including that for others and for oneself), *truthfulness* and *wisdom*. The idea of virtue as a balance between vices in relation to each of these can be helpful in thinking about the sort of person that one might want to be as a practitioner. Different commentators emphasize different lists of the virtues that they consider to be most important in the people professions. However, all point to the importance of being able to state the relationship between the individual and the professional community as a way of being explicit about which virtues should be considered to be important.

At the same time, it is very difficult for virtues to be codified. Modern professional communities are not as confined and able to be face-to-face as was the city-state of Athens in which Aristotle developed his ideas. The type of society in which modern professions have developed requires formal statements, by-laws to which third parties can refer and so on. For this reason, it can be difficult to incorporate virtue ethics into the *codes of ethics* and other documents that are now considered necessary. Yet, as Webb (2009) argues, virtue as an ethical concept is part of the everyday way in which practitioners consider their own and others' practice (compare with Pellegrino and Thomasma, 1993). The type of *wisdom* to which Aristotle referred as a virtue is the practical capacity to make good judgements and although codifying this quality is extremely difficult, practitioners can readily recognize it in those colleagues who demonstrate it throughout their work. This is the sort of colleague who others might wish to emulate. Such wisdom is likely to be seen in the ability to make good judgements not only about the technical matters with which practitioners are concerned but also in relation to the other virtues and the way that they both inform and can be displayed in practice. In this way, virtue ethics can contribute to the thinking and actions of practitioners in seeing to develop good practice.

KEY TEXTS
- Armstrong, A.E. *et al.* (2000) 'An Inquiry into Moral Virtues, Especially Compassion, in Psychiatric Nurses: Findings from a Delphi Study', *Journal of Psychiatric and Mental Health Nursing*, 7 (4): pp. 297–306

- Macallister, J. (2012) 'Virtue, Epistemology and the Philosophy of Education', *Journal of Philosophy of Education*, pp. 251–270
- Pellegrino, E.D. and Thomasma, D.C. (1993) *The Virtues in Medical Practice* (Oxford: Oxford University Press)
- Webb, S.A. (2009) 'Virtue Ethics' in M. Gray and S.A. Webb (eds), *Ethics and Value Perspectives in Social Work* (Basingstoke: Palgrave Macmillan)

W

welfare

SEE ALSO justice; politics; social justice; utilitarianism

The term welfare can have several different meanings in the people professions. First, it refers to the system of policies and institutional services that provide a 'social safety net'. This can include publicly funded health and education, personal care and income maintenance (social security). In this respect, it can mean the system within which a great deal of the activities of the people professions occur.

Second, the term welfare is used in a more restricted way to refer to one particular form of social security, namely, the provision of income support. This is found in the United States where 'welfare recipients' are those whose income includes direct cash transfers from government. This variation in terminology can provide the basis for the development of parallel debates and potential misapplication of ideas between settings in international comparative debates.

If taken as a broad set of ideas, these interpretations of welfare concern the institutional arrangements of advanced industrial societies to redress the lack of material means to a decent human life, at least at a minimally defined level. This generates particular ethical debates, concerning the relationship between *autonomy, beneficence, freedom* and *responsibility*. For example, is it *just* if one person is taxed in order to pay for another person to have an income or to receive education and health services? If so, what is a *fair* level in terms of the impact on the person paying tax and how well off the person receiving the transfer payments will be? The working lives of many members of the people professions are affected by the ways in which different countries answer these questions. In some areas of practice, such questions have an immediate significance, in that if education, health and social well-being are considered to be *rights*, then some means must be found to make them available. The level of services and the funding they receive is directly affected by the way societies answer this question.

However, what is to be done if the person who lacks welfare has in some way contributed to her or his own problem? An example that is widely used in these debates is of people who acquire life-threatening conditions that result from their own behaviour. The main sides of the argument are that from *utilitarianism* that tends to favour giving such a person lower priority when choices have to be made and that from *deontology* that tends to favour duties to each person on the clinical merit of their condition (see, e.g. Beauchamp and Childress, 2009, p. 263).

A third meaning of welfare is that of 'well-being' in the wider sense that is used by moral philosophers and that can also be understood as 'flourishing'. This is the idea that a definition of what is good must be found in those things that enable people to live good lives. However, within this understanding there are also debates about the ways in which well-being or flourishing can be understood and achieved. From some perspectives, such as *liberalism* and *utilitarianism*, the choice of those things that people regard as making a good life should be the free decision of the people concerned. From other points of view, such as *deontology, human rights* and *social justice,* it is not only possible but necessary to state what is required to live a decent human life. This is a form of what *pluralism* calls the incompatibility of values, in which freedom and equality are not easily reconciled. Indeed, the position taken by different commentators within this debate reveals the priority given to one or other of these *values* or the extent to which there is an attempt to find a balance.

An example of how this can appear in practice is that of a family with two parents and three children aged under 10 years, who have a relatively low income that includes some state social security payments. Their house has little furniture, they do not always pay their rent or their utility bills so that at times either the electricity or the water is disconnected. At the same time both parents smoke cigarettes and regularly drink alcohol. While there is no evidence of actual physical injury to the children, they do not always get meals. The question faced by practitioners (including medical practitioners, nurses, social workers, teachers and youth workers) is what is the right balance between the freedom of families to live as they choose and the imposition of standards of well-being that are determined from a professional perspective. In particular, in this situation, it is also relevant to consider whether the welfare of children over-rides the freedom of parents to make choices about their parenting: at what point does the widespread view that parents have the right to make such choices end – indeed, does it have a limit? Would the way this situation is seen change if the parents are identified as coming from an ethnic minority community that has a history of structural disadvantage?

This is precisely the situation facing members of these professions in Australia at the time of writing, in the implementation by the government of policies that quarantine social security payments to families and restrict what large parts of such payments can be spent on (Fawcett and Hanlon, 2009). These policies originally were not implemented universally, but in areas with predominantly Aboriginal populations. Within the people professions, as well as in the wider society, opinion is divided between those who consider that such a policy is bad (because it is discriminatory and does not address the underlying structural issues) and those who consider it good (because it has resulted in children being better fed, less domestic and family violence, lower incidences of problematic alcohol consumption and so on). So, from either side of this debate, it is clear that welfare is a highly complex value that involves many factors.

KEY TEXTS
- Adshead, G. and Sarkar, S.P. (2005) 'Justice and Welfare: Two Ethical Paradigms in Forensic Psychiatry', *Australian & New Zealand Journal of Psychiatry*, 39 (11/12): pp. 1011–1017
- Fawcett, B. and Hanlon, M. (2009) 'Child Sexual Abuse and Aboriginal Communities in Australia: A Case Study of Non-Inclusive Government Intervention', *European Journal of Social Work*, 12 (1): pp. 87–100
- Jecker, N.S. (2008) 'A Broader View of Justice', *American Journal of Bioethics*, 8 (10): pp. 2–10

whistle-blowing

SEE ALSO **loyalty; responsibility; supererogatory**

In situations where a practitioner considers that there has been malpractice or corruption, she or he may consider that it is necessary to report this outside the immediate work context in order that the situation might be redressed. This is known as 'whistle-blowing'. It may be done within an organization, for example, by disclosing information to senior colleagues about a wrong that has been observed elsewhere. Whistle-blowing also takes the form of people disclosing something wrong outside an organization, for example, by reporting it to government or to the press.

In a study of institutional care for adults with needs for assistance in daily living, Manthorpe and Stanley (1999) note that whistle-blowing is morally very complex. First, to be a morally good act, it must be based on the genuine belief that the actions that are being reported are breaches of ethical values and principles, not simply a disagreement about professional technique. Second, disclosure should be for the good of service users or of the wider service, not motivated by personal grievance. Third, while the person who discloses may consider duty to service users or the wider service to be of primary concern, others may regard the value of *loyalty* more highly or may think that the overall impact on service users or others outweighs the good that is achieved in making the matter public. Of course, in relation to this last point, some appeals to loyalty may be self-interested and against the interest of service users. The ethical point is that a decision to whistle blow is neither easy nor simple as it brings together elements of the ethics of *duty* and *responsibility* with *consequences*.

It cannot be assumed that even when it is widely accepted that a wrong has occurred and that disclosure enables this to be addressed that the whistle-blower will not then experience negative responses from others. There is a long history of people who have disclosed abuse or corruption then being subject to organizational sanctions, ostracism by other colleagues and so on. Indeed, it may not only be the perpetrator of an abuse or the whistle-blower who experiences such negative consequences, but also service users and colleagues. *Trust* may be considered very highly among some professional groups and the act of disclosure can be seen as a breach of this. However, Johnstone (1994) argues that in such circumstances this value is a matter of etiquette, in other words of 'good manners', rather than ethics as such and so is critical of practitioners who remain silent on abuse and corruption, as are Manthorpe and Stanley (1999).

Nevertheless, despite legislation in some jurisdictions that support the *rights* of whistle-blowers, it remains relatively high risk. There is more that organizations that employ people professions, including those that are owned and/or run by members of the professions, as well as professional bodies themselves could do to help practitioners identify appropriate strategies for responding to abuse and corruption and to provide support for those who make the principled judgement that whistle-blowing is the appropriate course of action. In the meantime, although the whistle-blower may be regarded by many people as doing the right thing, such an act is also often seen a *supererogatory* (i.e., above what can reasonably be expected of each and every member of the people professions as a basic ethical requirement).

KEY TEXTS

- Davis, A.J. and Konishi, E. (2007) 'Whistleblowing in Japan', *Nursing Ethics*, 14 (2): pp. 194–202
- De Maria, W. (1996) 'The Welfare Whistleblower: In Praise of Troublesome People', *Australian Social Work*, 49 (3): pp. 15–24
- Hooper, S. (2011) 'Understanding the Ethics of Whistleblowing by Nurses', *Journal of the Australian Rehabilitation Nurses Association*, 14 (3): pp. 18–21
- Jackson, D. *et al.* (2010) 'Understanding Whistleblowing: Qualitative Insights from Nurse Whistleblowers', *Journal of Advanced Nursing*, 66 (10): pp. 2194–2201

wisdom

SEE ALSO **phronesis; principles; trust; virtue**

Members of the people professions need to be able to know and do what is right in each specific situation that they face (Pellegrino and Thomasma, 1993). This capacity can be considered to be both a skill and a *virtue*. In that sense, it is a practical virtue that enables other virtues to be understood in their proper context. The ancient Greek philosopher Aristotle (384–322 BCE) wrote in terms of *phronesis*, which is best translated as 'practical wisdom'; in medieval Europe, it was also understood as 'prudence' (Hinman, 2012, p. 273). Hinman points out that there are two parts to this notion: practicality and sound judgement.

The first part of this notion, practicality, concerns the importance of being able to apply *values* and *principles*, which are quite general, to specific situations and events. To do so requires an understanding of both aspects (ideas and situations). While this is often enhanced through experience, so that wisdom is developed through practice, it does not emerge automatically. Nor is practicality to be understood only in cognitive terms. Rather, it combines cognition with emotional intelligence and intuition so that often a person who demonstrates this capacity may appear to 'have a feel for it', even if this comes after much reflection and learning through observation.

The second part of practical wisdom or prudence is that of sound judgement. It is not only that the person who demonstrates this capacity is capable of action but also that the action usually is focused accurately. The prudent person not only knows the best way of achieving a particular goal but also how to decide between goals in order to concentrate on those which are worth pursuing. Clearly this is not simply a matter of conforming to standard rules nor of seeking to please popular opinion. There may be times when prudent action does this, but it is also likely that in many situations it will not. For example, if we think that there are problems with the way in which an organization's policies are implemented, we may choose to challenge only those that we think are most important and about those it is worth having difficult conversations with colleagues.

As Hinman (2012, p. 276) also observes, practical wisdom is not only concerned with doing the right thing, such as telling the *truth*, but also of doing in a way that promotes human flourishing. The truth can be told in a way that confronts another person or undermines their integrity so that she or he then becomes unable to take in what is being said. The wise person finds a way of telling the truth so that it can be heard.

This notion of wisdom is congruent with a *pluralistic* approach to ethics. Not only is it important to be able to make sound judgements about the way in which general values and principles can inform each practice situation but in doing so of being able to grasp the insights of different ethical approaches. *Deontology* and *utilitarianism* provide very different frameworks for considering what is good and what is right, but each may have something valuable to contribute to making sound judgements and the balance between these may shift between particular situations. For example, when service users withhold their consent to interventions that the practitioner knows are the most likely to be helpful, it requires practical wisdom to know how best to attempt to gain the service users' *trust* sufficiently so that they listen carefully to professional advice. But it also requires practical wisdom to know when a refusal to consent to an intervention is reasonable even if the consequences appear to others to be unacceptable. Refusal to accept treatment in life-threatening medical situations is perhaps the instance that is most obvious, and indeed such circumstances do present medical, nursing and other health practitioners with serious ethical challenges.

Less immediate, but very serious in the long term, might be a refusal to accept other forms of assistance that would be profoundly beneficial for the service user, including assistance with parenting, with mental health problems and with the need for physical care in late life. Again, knowing when to press the point, perhaps because there is reason to think that the person lacks an accurate grasp of their problem or of the intervention being offered, and when to accept that the person's own values are such that she or he places greater weight on other aspects of the situation such as *autonomy* or of remaining in familiar surroundings even if that decreases autonomy and increases dependency in other ways. Or it may be that previous negative experiences of receiving assistance mean that service users do not accept further interventions. Being able to understand these responses and then possibly to continue to work with service users requires practical sound judgement.

The wise practitioner may not always be in agreement with colleagues, including those who may also be considered wise. This is inevitable and does not invalidate the view that they demonstrate wisdom. In a world of plural values, this is to be expected. What matters is that over time such practitioners show that they are able to bring together values and principles to make sound judgements and through this to demonstrate good practice.

KEY TEXTS
- Bondi, L. *et al.* (eds) (2011) *Towards Professional Wisdom* (Farnham: Ashgate)

- Pellegrino, E.D. and Thomasma, D.C. (1993) *The Virtues in Medical Practice* (Oxford: Oxford University Press)
- Sellman, D. (2009) 'Practical Wisdom in Health and Social Care: Teaching for Professional Phronesis', *Learning in Health and Social Care*, 8 (2): pp. 84–91
- Tsang, (2008) 'Kairos and Practice Wisdom in Social Work Practice', *European Journal of Social Work*, 11 (2): pp. 131–143
- Uhrenfeldt, L. and Hall, E.O.C. (2007) 'Clinical Wisdom among Proficient Nurses', *Nursing Ethics*, 14 (3): pp. 397–398
- Widdershoven, G. *et al.* (2009) 'Empirical Ethics as Dialogic Practice', *Bioethics*, 23 (4): pp. 236–248

further reading

At the end of keyword entry, I have recommended some selected further readings in relation to the specific topic. For the reader who is interested to know more in depth about ethical discussions related to particular professions more generally, the following readings are suggested. They are selected from recent writing about professional ethics. Journal recommendations concentrate on ethics-specific publications, although many other professional journals may contain some articles on ethics. Some texts that others find useful may be omitted here; these notes are not intended to be exhaustive but to indicate core material.

General

There are relatively few books that address the 'caring', 'helping' or 'people' professions generally and as a whole. The author has written about the contribution of recent debates in ethical theory to these professions, looking at emotions, relationships and care; ecological ethics and postmodern ethics in: Hugman, R. (2005) *New Approaches in Ethics for the Caring Professions* (Basingstoke: Palgrave Macmillan). A recent collection that discusses various professions is: Bondi, L., Carr, D., Clark, C. and Clegg, C. (eds) (2011) *Towards Professional Wisdom: Practical Deliberations in the People Professions* (Aldershot: Ashgate), which has chapters on teaching, social work, psychotherapy, religious ministry and allied health, as well as some general discussions of concepts including that of 'wisdom'. An innovative approach is provided by: Koehn, D. (1994) *The Ground of Professional Ethics* (London: Routledge). She proposes a particular view of professionalism as an expression of ethical ideals. In addition: Banks, S. and Gallagher, A. (2009) *Ethics in Professional Life: Virtues for Health and Social Care* (Basingstoke: Palgrave Macmillan) focuses on the virtues in professional practice. The journal *Professional Ethics* was incorporated into *Business & Professional Ethics* from 2004, and this continues to carry articles related to these professions both generally and specifically.

Allied health

One of the most influential books in this area is: Veatch, R.M. and Flack, H. (1997) *Case Studies in Allied Health Ethics* (Prentice Hall). It remains one of the few to address the allied health professions (or remedial therapies) together. More recent material that examines particular professions within this group include: Gabbard, D.L. and Martin, M.W. (2010) *Physical Therapy Ethics*. 2nd edn (Philadelphia, PA: F.A. Davis Company), which considers the questions of professionalism and practice issues and examines cultural diversity. This book may also be of interest to occupational therapists. Complementing these other references, from a slightly different perspective, is: Body, R. and McAllister, L. (2009) *Ethics in Speech and Language Therapy* (Chichester: Wiley-Blackwell). This book argues clearly for a notion of healthcare ethics, linking speech and language therapy to other allied health professions, while focusing specifically on speech pathology issues.

Medicine (and biomedical ethics)

While there are many textbooks on medical and biomedical ethics, probably the most influential work in this field is: Beauchamp, T. and Childress, J. (2009) *Principles of Biomedical Ethics*. 6th edn (New York: Oxford University Press). Originally published in 1979, this work has developed along with thinking in this field. Although lengthy and detailed, this book contains very clear examples of how different concepts and principles apply to practice in the field of health. In addition, particularly influential in biomedical ethics has been: Pellegrino, E.D. and Thomasma, D.C. (1993) *The Virtues in Medical Practice* (Oxford: Oxford University Press). DeGrazia, D., Mappes, T.A. and Brand-Ballard, J. (eds) (2010) *Biomedical Ethics* (New York: McGraw-Hill) contains a range of chapters by practitioners and academics looking at principles and concepts in relation to clinical challenges. Likewise, a wide range of views including work from leading ethicists is included in: Kuhse, H. and Singer, P. (eds) *A Companion to Bioethics*. 2nd edn (Oxford: Blackwell). The *Journal of Medical Ethics* is the premier source of current articles in this area, and is published in the United Kingdom by the *British Medical Journal* group.

Nursing

There are several leading references in nursing. Tschudin, V. (2003) *Ethics in Nursing: The Caring Relationship.* 3rd edn (Oxford: Butterworth-Heinemann) emphasizes the professionalism of nursing and focuses on questions of care (including the ethics of care) and professional virtues. It contains several chapters on practice issues. Fry, S.T. and Johnstone, M.-J. (2002) *Ethics in Nursing Practice.* 2nd edn (Oxford: Blackwell) structures a discussion of principles and concepts around an applied view of the nursing role. Thompson, I.E., Melia, K.M. and Boyd, K.M. (2000) *Nursing Ethics.* 4th edn (London: Churchill Livingstone). The textbook covers all the major issues very clearly. It begins by looking at individual practice and then broadens out to examine organizational contexts and health policies. Another text by leading nursing ethics writers is: Fry, S.T., Veatch, R.M. and Taylor, C. (2010) *Case Studies in Nursing Ethics.* 4th edn (Sudbury, MA: Jones & Bartlett). This book looks at the core biomedical concepts and then applies these to a range of practice situations. The major international journal in this area is *Nursing Ethics.*

Psychology and psychotherapy

Although the underlying principles and concepts are very similar, in psychology discussions of ethics these are greatly influenced by different institutional contexts of practice and national codes of ethics. A thorough coverage in this field from the United States is provided by: Koocher, G.P. and Keith-Spiegel, P. (2008) *Ethics in Psychology and the Mental Health Professions: Standards and Cases.* 2nd edn (New York: Oxford University Press). It focuses especially on clinical relationships and professional virtues. In the United Kingdom, Francis, R.D. (2009) *Ethics for Psychologists.* 2nd edn (Chichester: Blackwell Publishers) presents a textbook that considers ethics in practice. This looks in detail at practical challenges; it also includes a discussion of human rights with reference to the *Universal Convention* (UN, 1948). Truscott, D. and Crook, K.H. (2004) *Ethics for the Practice of Psychology in Canada* (Edmonton: University of Alberta Press) examines principles, standards, decision-making and also some specific issues such as that of consent. Probably one of the most widely used texts in psychotherapy ethics is: Corey, G., Corey, M.S. and Callanan, P. (2011) *Issues and Ethics in the Helping Professions*. 11th edn (Belmont, CA: Brooks/Cole), which, despite the breadth of its title, focuses quite explicitly and very thoroughly on counselling and psychotherapy.

Social work and human services
In social work and human services, one of the most comprehensive discussion is provided by: Banks, S. (2012) *Ethics and Values in Social Work*. 4th edn (Basingstoke: Palgrave Macmillan). This book clearly explains all the major approaches to ethics and the way in which these relate to practice. The same author looks in depth at practitioners' views of how they deal with ethical challenges in: Banks, S. (2004) *Ethics, Accountability and the Social Professions* (Basingstoke: Palgrave Macmillan). In the United States, an influential text is: Reamer, F.G. (2006) *Social Work Values and Ethics*. 3rd edn (New York: Columbia University Press), which includes a detailed discussion of risk management in ethical matters. Another that looks at ethics in decision-making is: Dolgoff, R., Harrington, D. and Loewenberg, F.M. (2011) *Ethical Decisions for Social Work Practice*. 9th edn (Belmont, CA: Brooks/Cole). Also worth looking at are: Congress, E. P. (1999) *Social Work Values and Ethics: Identifying and Resolving Professional Dilemmas* (Nelson Hall), which presents a decision-making model; Beckett, C. and Maynard, A. (2005) *Values and Ethics in Social Work: An Introduction* (London: Sage Publications), which is, as it says, an introductory text; and Bowles, W., Collingridge, M., Curry, S. and Valentine, B. (2006) *Ethical Practice in Social Work: An Applied Approach* (St Leonards, NSW: Allen & Unwin), which is an Australian text that, as its title suggests, demonstrates how ethical concepts can be applied to thinking about practice. The ethical dimension of the issue of anti-oppressive practice, which is increasingly important in critical approaches to social work, is explored in detail in: Clifford, D. and Burke, B. (2009) *Anti-Oppressive Ethics and Values in Social Work* (Basingstoke: Palgrave Macmillan). A recently launched journal, *Ethics & Social Welfare*, covers many aspects of social work and human services.

Teaching

A key book in the field of teaching is: Carr, D. (2000) *Professionalism and Ethics in Teaching* (London: Routledge). It explores the ethics of professionalism and teaching theory as well as practice in schools; it also discusses the meaning of professionalism for school teachers in ethical terms. Taking a slightly different approach is: Strike, K.A. and Soltis, J.F. (2004) *The Ethics of Teaching*. 4th edn (New York: Teachers College Press). This textbook examines the ethical issues of school teaching through the lens of classroom practice. A similar way of examining professional ethics can be found in: Keith-Spiegel, P., Whitley, B.J., Balogh, D.W., Perkins, D.V. and Wittig, A.F. (2002) *The Ethics of Teaching: A Casebook*. 2nd edn (Mahwah, NJ: Lawrence Erlbaum Associates Inc.), which focuses on the detail of practice in teaching, both in the classroom and in the wider school situation, using short discussions of everyday issues. In their introduction, they comment on the historical lack of material on ethics in teaching and this is reflected in that there is no identifiable specialist journal in this aspect of educational practice.

Youth work

As with teaching, writing about ethics in the field of youth work has quite a short history. A major text in this area is: Sercombe, H. (2010) *Youth Work Ethics* (London: Sage Publications). This is a very thorough examination of principles and concepts, linked to a very clear discussion of how these apply in practice. It offers a strong service user-centred approach to the ethics of youth work. Banks, S. (ed) (2010) *Ethical Issues in Youth Work* (London: Routledge) contains a range of chapters by different contributors. It is divided into two parts – the contexts of youth work and issues in practice. In both respect, the discussions are clear and detailed, presenting concepts through an understanding of how practice actually occurs. The same applied approach is also found in: Roberts, J. (2009) *Youth Work Ethics: Empowering Youth and Community Work Practice* (London: Learning Matters). This text book provides a very accessible style, with an overview of detailed practical considerations.

references

Adams, R. (2008) *Empowerment, Participation and Social Work* (Basingstoke: Palgrave Macmillan)

Adshead, G. and Sarkar, S.P. (2005) 'Justice and Welfare: Two Ethical Paradigms in Forensic Psychiatry', *Australian & New Zealand Journal of Psychiatry*, 39 (11/12): pp. 1011–1017

Allen, J.G. (2007) 'Evil, Mindblindness and Trauma: Challenges to Hope', *Smith College Studies in Social Work*, 77 (1): pp. 9–31

Allmark, P. (1995) 'Can There Be an Ethics of Care?' *Journal of Medical Ethics*, 21 (1): pp. 19–24

Annan, K. (1997) 'Ignorance Not Knowledge... Makes Enemies of Man', *UNHCRH*. Electronic document, downloaded on 21 September 2010 from http://www.unhchr.ch/huricane/huricane.nsf/view01/EF16892B 9B9D46ABC125662E00352F63?opendocument>

Armstrong, A.E., Parsons, S. and Barker, P.J. (2000) 'An Inquiry into Moral Virtues, Especially Compassion, in Psychiatric Nurses: Findings from a Delphi Study', *Journal of Psychiatric and Mental Health Nursing*, 7 (4): pp. 297–306

Arnd-Caddigan, M. and Pozzuto, R. (2009) 'The Virtuous Social Worker: The Role of "Thirdness" in Ethical Decision Making', *Families in Society: The Journal of Contemporary Social Services*, 90 (3): pp. 32332–32338

Aube, N. (2011) 'Ethical Challenges for Psychologists Doing Humanitarian Work', *Canadian Psychologist*, 52 (3): pp. 225–229

Banks, S. (2004) *Ethics, Accountability and the Social Professions* (Basingstoke Palgrave Macmillan)

Banks, S. (2012) *Ethics and Values in Social Work*. 4th edn (Basingstoke: Palgrave Macmillan)

Bauman, Z. (1993) *Postmodern Ethics* (Oxford: Blackwell)

Bauman, Z. (2001) *The Individualized Society* (Cambridge: Polity Press)

Beauchamp, T.L. and Childress, J.F. (2009) *Principles of Biomedical Ethics*. 6th edn (New York: Oxford University Press)

Begley, A.M. (2008) 'Truth-Telling, Honesty and Compassion: A Virtue-Based Exploration of a Dilemma in Practice', *International Journal of Nursing Practice*, 14 (5): pp. 336–341

Bennett, B. *et al.*, (eds) (2012) *Our Voices* (South Yarra VIC: Palgrave Macmillan)

Berlin, I. (1968) *Four Essays on Liberty* (Oxford: Oxford University Press)

Besthorn, F.H. (2002) 'Radical Environmentalism and the Ecological Self: Rethinking the Concept of Self-Identity for Social Work Practice', *Journal of Progressive Human Services*, 13 (1): pp. 53–72

Biestek, F.P. (1959) *The Casework Relationship* (London: George Allen & Unwin)

Bondi, L. *et al.*, (eds) (2011) *Towards Professional Wisdom: Practical Deliberations in the People Professions* (Farnham: Ashgate)

Bowles, W. *et al.*, (2006) *Ethical Practice in Social Work: An Applied Approach* (St Leonards, NSW: Allen & Unwin)

Botes, A. (1999) 'Nursing Ethics in a Developing Country', *Curationis*, 22 (1): pp. 64–67

Bradshaw, A. (1996) 'Yes! There Is an Ethics of Care: An Answer for Peter Allmark', *Journal of Medical Ethics*, 22 (1): pp. 8–12

Brameld, K.J. and Holman, C.D.J. (2005) 'The Use of End-Quintile Comparisons to Identify Under-Servicing of the Poor and Over-Servicing of the Rich: A Longitudinal Study Describing the Effect of Socioeconomic Status on Healthcare', *BMC Health Services Research*, 5: p. 61 [electronic journal, accessed on 24/9/2012 from http://www.ncbi.nlm.nih.gov/pmc/articles/PMC1236924/]

Bransford, C.L. (2011) 'Reconciling Paternalism and Empowerment in Clinical Practice: An Intersubjective Perspective', *Social Work*, 56 (1): pp. 36–42

Braveman, P.A. *et al.*, (2011) 'Health Disparities and Health Equity: The Issue Is Justice', *American Journal of Public Health*, 101 (Supplement 1): pp. S149–S155

Brown, M.B. (2011) 'Three Ways to Politicize Bioethics', *American Journal of Bioethics*, 9 (2): pp. 42–53

Browne, A.J. (1995) 'The Meaning of Respect: A First Nations' Perspective', *Canadian Journal of Nursing Research*, 27 (4): pp. 95–110

Burks, D.J. and Kobus, A.M. (2012) 'The Legacy of Altruism in Health Care: The Promotion of Empathy, Prosociality and Humanism', *Medical Education*, 46 (3): pp. 317–325

Butcher, H. *et al.*, (2007) *Critical Community Practice* (Bristol: Policy Press)

Carlisle, D. (2010) 'Beyond the Call of Duty: Physiotherapists Do Not Have to Be at the Top of Organisations to Effect Considerable Improvements in Patient Care', *Frontline*, 16 (11): pp. 20–22

Carr, D. (2000) *Professionalism and Ethics in Teaching* (London: Routledge)

Clancy, A. and Svensson, T. (2007) '"Faced" with Responsibility: Levinasian Ethics and the Challenge of Responsibility in Norwegian Public Health Nursing', *Nursing Philosophy*, 8 (3): pp. 158–166

Clark, P.G., Cott, C. and Drinka, T.J.K. (2007) 'Theory and Practice in Interprofessional Ethics: A Framework for Understanding Ethical Issues in Healthcare Teams', *Journal of Interprofessional Care*, 21 (6): pp. 591–603

Clifford, D. and Burke, B. (2009) *Anti-Oppressive Ethics and Values in Social Work* (Basingstoke: Palgrave Macmillan)

Collingridge, M., Miller, S. and Bowles, W. (2001) 'Privacy and Confidentiality in Social Work', *Australian Social Work*, 54 (2): pp. 3–13

Corneau, S. and Stergiopoulos, V. (2012) 'More Than Being against It: Anti-Racism and Anti-Oppression in Mental Health', *Journal of Transcultural Psychiatry*, 49 (2): pp. 261–282

Crewe, S.E. (2004) 'A Time to Be Silent and a Time to Speak Up', *Reflections: Narratives of Professional Helping*, 10 (1): pp. 16–25

Crigger, N.J. (2008) 'Towards a Viable and Just Global Ethics of Nursing', *Nursing Ethics*, 15 (1): pp. 17–27

Crigger, N.J. (2010) 'Towards Understanding the Nature of Conflict of Interest and Its Application to the Discipline of Nursing', *Nursing Philosophy*, 10 (4): pp. 253–262

Curren, R. (ed) 'Symposium on Sentimentalist Moral Education', *Theory and Research in Education*, 8 (2): pp. 123–197

Daly, L.K. (2012) 'Slaves Immersed in a Liberal Ideology', *Nursing Philosophy*, 13 (1): pp. 69–77

Davidhizar, R. (2005) 'Benevolent Power', *Journal of Practical Nursing*, 55 (4): pp. 5–9

Davis, A.J. and Konishi, E. (2007) 'Whistleblowing in Japan', *Nursing Ethics*, 14 (2): pp. 194–202

De Maria, W. (1996) 'The Welfare Whistleblower: In Praise of Troublesome People', *Australian Social Work*, 49 (3): pp. 15–24

de Vries, M.C. and Verhagen, A.A.E. (2008) 'The Case against Something That Is Not the Case', *American Journal of Bioethics*, 8 (11): pp. 29–31

Dean, E. (2001) 'Neo-Confucianism and Physiotherapy: The Mind-Body-Spirit Connection', *Hong Kong Physiotherapy Journal*, 19, pp. 3–8

DeFillipis, J. (2009) 'What's Left in the Community? Oppositional Politics in Contemporary Practice', *Community Development Journal*, 44 (1): pp. 38–52

Degner, L.F. (2002) 'Discourse, Ethics and Decision-making: Lessons from the Cancer Wars', *Canadian Journal of Nursing Research*, 34 (3): pp. 9–13

Dickinson, S.M.D. (1995) 'Beyond the Call of Duty: Memoirs of a Nurse in Hiroshima ... Excepts from Misako's Writings from 1979', *Journal of Practical Nursing*, 45 (2): pp. 23–26

Dinç, L. and Gastmans, C. (2012) 'Trust and Trustworthiness in Nursing: An Argument-Based Literature Review', *Nursing Inquiry*, 19 (3): pp. 223–237

Dodd, S.J. (2007) 'Identifying the Discomfort: An Examination of Ethical Issues Encountered by MSW Students during Field Placement', *Journal of Teaching in Social Work*, 27 (1): pp. 1–19

Dong, D. and Temple, B. (2011) 'Oppression: A Concept Analysis and Implications for Nursing and Nurses', *Nursing Forum*, 46 (3): pp. 169–176

Dwyer, J. (2009) 'How to Connect Bioethics and Environmental Ethics: Health, Sustainability, and Justice', *Bioethics*, 23 (9): pp. 497–502

Edwards, I. *et al.*, (2011) 'New Perspectives on the Theory of Justice: Implications for Physical Therapy Ethics and Clinical Practice', *Physical Therapy*, 91 (11): pp. 1642–1652

Edwards, S.D. (2011) 'Is There a Distinctive Ethics of Care?' *Nursing Ethics*, 18 (2): pp. 184–191

Emmerich, N. (2011) 'Whatever Happened to Medical Politics?' *Journal of Medical Ethics*, 37 (10): pp. 631–636

England, H. (1983) *Social Work as Art* (Hemel Hempstead: Allen & Unwin)

Englund, T. (2011) 'The Potential of Education for Creating Mutual Trust: Schools as Sites for Deliberation', *Educational Philosophy and Theory*, 43 (3): pp. 236–248

Epright, M.C. (2010) 'Coercing Future Freedom: Consent and Capacities for Autonomous Choice', *Journal of Law, Medicine and Ethics*, 38 (4): pp. 799–806

Epstein, I. (2009) 'Promoting Harmony Where There Is Commonly Conflict', *Social Work in Health Care*, 48 (3): pp. 216–231

Epstein, M. (2011) 'If I Were a Rich Man Could I Sell a Pancreas? A Study in the Locus of Oppression', *Journal of Medical Ethics*, 37 (2): pp. 109–112

Erlingsson, C.L. (2011) 'Evil and Elder Abuse', *Nursing Philosophy*, 12 (4): pp. 248–261

Fawcett, B. and Hanlon, M. (2009) 'Child Sexual Abuse and Aboriginal Communities in Australia: A Case Study of Non-inclusive Government Intervention', *European Journal of Social Work*, 12 (1): pp. 87–100

Ferguson, E., Farrell, K. and Lawrence, C. (2008) 'Blood Donation as an Act of Benevolence Rather Than Altruism', *Health Psychology*, 27 (3): pp. 27–36

Frankena, W. (1973) *Ethics*. 2nd edn (Englewood Cliffs, NJ: Prentice Hall)

Freeman, S.J. (2000) *Ethics: An Introduction to Philosophy and Practice* (Belmont CA: Wadsworth)

Freidson, E. (2001) *Professionalism: The Third Logic* (Chicago: University of Chicago Press)

Fry, S. and Johnstone, M.-J. (2002) *Ethics in Nursing Practice*. 2nd edn (Oxford: Blackwell)

Fry, S., Veatch, R.M. and Taylor, C. (2010) *Case Studies in Nursing Ethics.* 4th edn (Sudbury, MA: Jones & Bartlett)

Fulcher, L. and McGladdery, S. (2011) 'Re-examining Social Work Roles and Tasks with Foster Care', *Child & Youth Services*, 32 (10): pp. 19–38

Gabel, S. (2011) 'Ethics and Values in Clinical Practice: Whom Do They Help?' *Mayo Clinic Proceedings*, 86 (5): pp. 421–424

Gadow, S. (1999) 'Relational Narrative: The Postmodern Turn in Nursing Ethics', *Scholarly Inquiry for Nursing Practice*, 13 (1): pp. 57–70

Gallagher, (1999) 'The Ethics of Compassion', *Ostomy/Wound Management*, 45 (6): pp. 14–16

Gauthier, J. (2009) 'Ethical Principles and Human Rights: Building a Better World Globally', *Counselling Psychology Quarterly*, 22 (1): pp. 25–32

Geisinger, J. (2012) 'Respect in Education', *Journal of Philosophy of Education*, 46 (1): pp. 110–112

Gilligan, C. (1982) *In a Different Voice* (Cambridge, MA: Harvard University Press)

Gilligan, P. and Akhtar, S. (2006) 'Cultural Barriers in the Disclosure of Child Sexual Abuse in Asian Communities: Listening to What Women Say', *British Journal of Social Work*, 36 (8): pp. 1361–1377

Girod, J. and Beckman, A.W. (2005) 'Just Allocation and Team Loyalty: A New Virtue Ethic for Emergency Medicine', *Journal of Medical Ethics*, 31 (10): pp. 567–570

Glannon, W. and Ross, L.F. (2002) 'Are Doctors Altruistic?' *Journal of Medical Ethics*, 28 (2): pp. 69–69

Good, H. (2004) 'Honor role', *Teacher Magazine*, 16 (2): pp. 46–48

Gostin, L.O. (2004) 'Health of the People: The Highest Law?' *Journal of Law, Medicine and Ethics*, 32 (3): pp. 509–515

Gournay, K. (1998) 'Ethical Issues in Mental Health Nursing' in W. Tadd (ed), *Ethical Issues in Nursing and Midwifery Practice* (Basingstoke: Macmillan)

Gower, B.S. (1992) 'What Do We Owe Future Generations?' in D.E. Cooper and J.A. Palmer (eds), *The Environment in Question: Ethics and Global Issues* (Buckingham: Open University Press)

Graham, M. (2002) *Social Work and African-Centred World Views* (Birmingham: Venture Press)

Gray, J. (1996) *After Social Democracy* (London: Demos)

Gray, M. (2010) 'Postmodern Ethics' in M. Gray and S.A. Webb (eds), *Ethics and Value Perspectives in Social Work* (Basingstoke: Palgrave Macmillan)

Habermas, J. (1990) *Moral Consciousness and Communicative Action.* (Trans. C. Lenhardt and S.W. Nicholsen) (Cambridge, MA: MIT Press)

Halifax, J. (2012) 'A Heuristic Model of Enactive Compassion', *Current Opinion in Supportive and Palliative Care*, 6 (2): pp. 228–235

Häyry, M. (2005) 'A Defense of Ethical Relativism', *Cambridge Quarterly of Healthcare Ethics*, 14 (1): pp. 7–12

Hawkins, R., Redley, M. and Hooland, A.J. (2011) 'Duty of Care and Autonomy: How Support Workers Managed the Tension between Protecting Service Users from Risk and Promoting Their Independence in a Specialist Group Home', *Journal of Intellectual Disability Research*, 55 (9): pp. 873–884

Healy, L.M. (2007) 'Universalism and Cultural Relativism in Social Work Ethics', *International Social Work*, 50 (1): pp. 11–26

Held, V. (1993) *Feminist Morality* (Chicago: University of Chicago Press)

Helm, C.M. (2006) 'Teacher Dispositions as Predictors of Good Teaching', *Clearing House: A Journal of Educational Strategies*, 79 (3): pp. 117–118

Hess, J.D. (2003) 'Gadow's Relational Narrative: An Elaboration', *Nursing Philosophy*, 4 (2): pp. 137–148

Hinman, L.H. (2012) *Ethics: A Pluralistic Approach to Moral Theory*. 5th edn (Boston, MA: Wadsworth)

Hoagland, S.L. (1996) 'Lesbian Ethics and Female Agency', *Journal of Lesbian Studies*, 1 (2): pp. 195–208

Hodge, D.R., Limb, G.E. and Cross, T.L. (2009) 'Moving from Colonization to Balance and Harmony: A Native American Perspective on Wellness', *Social Work*, 54 (3): pp. 211–219

Holloway, M. (2007) 'Spiritual Need and the Core Business of Social Work', *British Journal of Social Work*, 37 (2): pp. 265–280

Hooper, S. (2011) 'Understanding the Ethics of Whistleblowing by Nurses', *Journal of the Australian Rehabilitation Nurses Association*, 14 (3): pp. 18–21

Houston, S. (2001) 'Transcending the Fissure in Risk Theory: Critical Realism and Child Welfare', *Child and Family Social Work*, 6 (3): pp. 219–228

Houston, S. (2010) 'Discourse Ethics' in M. Gray and S.A. Webb (eds), *Ethics and Value Perspectives in Social Work* (Basingstoke: Palgrave Macmillan)

Hugaas, J.V. (2010) 'Evil's Place in the Ethics of Social Work', *Ethics & Social Welfare*, 4 (3): pp. 254–279

Hughes Tuohey, C. (2012) 'Reform and the Politics of Hybridization in Mature Health Care States', *Journal of Health Politics, Policy and Law*, 37 (4): pp. 611–632

Hugman, R. (1991) *Power in Caring Professions* (Basingstoke: Macmillan – now Palgrave Macmillan)

Hugman, R. (1998) *Social Welfare and Social Value* (Basingstoke: Macmillan – now Palgrave Macmillan)

Hugman, R. (2003) 'Professional Values and Ethics in Social Work: Reconsidering Postmodernism?' *British Journal of Social Work*, 33 (8): pp. 1025–1041

Hugman, R. (2005) *New Approaches in Ethics for the Caring Professions* (Basingstoke: Palgrave Macmillan)

Hugman, R. (2013) *Culture, Values and Ethics in Social Work* (London: Routledge)

Huong, D.B. *et al.*, (2007) 'Rural Health Care in Vietnam and China: Conflict between Market Reforms and Social Need', *International Journal of Health Services*, 37 (3): pp. 555–572

Husband, C. (1995) 'The Morally Active Practitioner and the Ethics of Anti-Racist Social Work' in R. Hugman and D. Smith (eds), *Ethical Issues in Social Work* (London: Routledge)

Hyun, I. (2008) 'Clinical Cultural Competence and the Threat of Ethical Relativism', *Cambridge Quarterly of Healthcare Ethics*, 17 (2): pp. 154–163

Ife, J. (2012) *Human Rights and Social Work*. 3rd edn (Melbourne: Cambridge University Press)

International Council of Nursing [ICN] (2006) *The ICN Code of Ethics for Nurses* (Geneva: ICN)

International Federation of Social Workers [IFSW]/International Association of Schools of Social Work [IASSW] (2004) *Ethics in Social Work: Statement of Principles* [electronic document, http://www.ifsw.org/f38000032.html, date accessed 1/2/2011]

International Union of Psychological Science [IUPS] (2008) *Universal Declaration of Ethical Principles for Psychologists*, http://www.iupsys.net/index.php/ethics/declaration [date accessed 23/2/2011]

Irvine, R. *et al.*, (2002) 'Interprofessionalism and Ethics: Consensus or Clash of Cultures?' *Journal of Interprofessional Care*, 16 (3): pp. 199–210

Jackson, *et al.*, (2010) 'Understanding Whistleblowing: Qualitative Insights from Nurse Whistleblowers', *Journal of Advanced Nursing*, 66 (10): pp. 2194–2201

Jaggar, A. (1992) 'Feminist Ethics' in L. Becker and C. Becker (eds), *Encyclopedia of Ethics* (New York: Garland Press)

Jecker, N.S. (2008) 'A Broader View of Justice', *American Journal of Bioethics*, 8 (10): pp. 2–10

Jecker, N.S. and Self, D.J. (1991) 'Separating Care and Cure: An Analysis of Historical and Contemporary Images of Nursing and Medicine', *Journal of Medicine and Philosophy*, 16 (3): pp. 285–306

Johnstone, M.-J. (2011) 'Nursing and Justice as a Basic Human Need', *Nursing Philosophy*, 12 (1): pp. 34–44

Johnstone, M.-J. (2011) 'Choice and Human Freedom', *Australian Nursing Journal*, 19 (3): p. 22

Johnstone, M.-J. (1994) *Bioethics: A Nursing Perspective* (Marrickville, NSW: W.B. Saunders/Baillière-Tindall)

Kangasniemi, M. (2010) 'Equality as a Central Concept of Nursing Ethics', *Scandinavian Journal of Caring Sciences*, 24 (4): pp. 824–832

Kant, I. (1991 [1785]) *Groundwork of the Metaphysic of Morals* (ed, H.J. Paton) (London: Routledge)

Kaplan, L.E. (2009) 'A Conceptual Framework for Considering Informed Consent', *Journal of Social Work Ethics and Values*, 6 (3) (on-line journal, available at http://www.socialworker.com/jswve/content/view/130/69/)

Karenga, M. (2004) *Maat: The Moral Ideal in Ancient Egypt. A Study in Classical African Ethics* (London: Routledge)

Karlsen, J.R. and Solbakk, J.H. (2011) 'A Waste of Time: The Problem of Common Morality in *Principles of Biomedical Ethics*', *Journal of Medical Ethics*, 37 (1): pp. 588–591

Kekes, J. (1993) *The Morality of Pluralism* (Princeton, NJ: Princeton University Press)

Killmister, S. (2010) 'Dignity, Not Such a Useless Concept', *Journal of Medical Ethics*, 36 (3): pp. 160–164

Kirby, J. (2010) 'Enhancing the Fairness of Pandemic Critical Care Triage', *Journal of Medical Ethics*, 36 (12): pp. 758–761

Kirsch, N.R. (20) 'Unsatisfying Satisfaction', *PT in Motion*, 2 (8): pp. 44–46

Kittay, E.F. (1999) *Love's Labors: Essays on Women, Equality and Dependency* (New York: Routledge)

Koehn, D. (1994) *The Ground of Professional Ethics* (London: Routledge)

Koh, E. and Koh, C. (2008) 'Caring for Older Adults: The Parables in Confucian Texts', *Nursing Science Quarterly*, 21 (4): pp. 365–368

Konishi, E., Yahiro, M., Nakajima, N. and Ono, M. (2009) 'The Japanese Value of Harmony and Nursing Ethics', *Nursing Ethics*, 16 (5): pp. 625–636

Kuhse, H. (1997) *Caring, Nurses, Women and Ethics* (Oxford: Blackwell)

Kunyk, D. and Austin, W. (2012) 'Nursing under the Influence: A Relational Ethics Perspective', *Nursing Ethics*, 19 (3): pp. 380–389

Kymlicka, W. (1989) *Liberalism, Community and Culture* (Oxford: The Clarendon Press)

Lai, K. (2006) *Learning From Chinese Philosophies: Ethics of Interdependent and Contextualised Self* (Aldershot: Ashgate)

Le Granse, M., Kinébanian, A. and Josephsson, S. (2006) 'Promoting Autonomy of the Client with Persistent Mental Illness', *Occupational Therapy International*, 13 (3): pp. 142–159

Leget, C. and Olthuis, G. (2007) 'Compassion as a Basis for Ethics in Medical Education', *Journal of Medical Ethics*, 33 (10): pp. 617–620

Lindh, I. *et al.*, (2010) 'Courage and Nursing Practice a Theoretical Analysis', *Nursing Ethics*, 17 (5): pp. 551–565

Liu, W.T. and Kendig, H. (eds) (2000) *Who Should Care for the Elderly? An East-West Value Divide* (Singapore: Singapore University Press/World Scientific Publishing Co. Pte. Ltd.)

Loewy, E.H. and Loewy, R.S. (2004) *Textbook of Healthcare Ethics*. 2nd edn (Dordrecht: Kluwer)

Macallister, J. (2012) 'Virtue, Epistemology and the Philosophy of Education', *Journal of Philosophy of Education*, pp. 251–270

MacIntye, A. (1998) *A Short History of Ethics* (London: Routedge)

Macklin, R. (2003) 'Dignity Is a Useless Concept', *British Medical Journal*, 327 (7429): pp. 1419–1420

Majmudar, U. (2005) *Gandhi's Pilgrimage of Faith: From Darkness to Light* (Albany: State University of New York Press)

Malaudzi, F.M., Libster, M.M. and Phiri, S. (2009) 'Suggestions for Creating a Welcoming Nursing Community: Ubuntu, Cultural Diplomacy and Mentoring', *International Journal for Human Caring*, 13 (2): pp. 45–51

Manthorpe, J. and Stanley, N. (1999) 'Shifting the Focus from "Bad Apples" to Users' Rights' in N. Stanley, J. Manthorpe and B. Penhale (eds), *Institutional Abuse* (London: Routledge)

Maslow, A. (1954) *Motivation and Personality* (New York: Harper)

Mayville, K.L. (2011) 'Technology, Cheating, Ethics, and Strategies for Creating a Culture of Honesty', *Chart*, 109 (3): pp. 6–10

Mbiti, J.S. (1990) *African Religions and Philosophy*. 2nd edn (Oxford: Heinemann Educational Publishers)

McCleland, A. (2011) 'Culturally Safe Nursing Research: Exploring the Use of an Indigenous Research Methodology from an Indigenous Researcher's Perspective', *Journal of Transcultural Nursing*, 22 (4): pp. 362–367

McKinnon, J. (2008) 'Exploring the Nexus between Social Work and the Environment', *Australian Social Work*, 61 (3): pp. 256–268

Medrum, H. (2011) 'Spirituality in Medical Practice: How Humanitarian Physicians Draw Their Boundaries with Patients', *Integrative Medicine: A Clinician's Journal*, 10 (3). pp. 26–30

Meiers, S.J. and Bauer, D.J. (2008) 'Existential Caring in the Family Health Experience', *Scandinavian Journal of Caring Sciences*, 22 (1): pp. 110–117

Midgley, M. (2001) *Gaia: The Next Big Idea* (London: Demos)

Mji, G. *et al.*, (2011) 'An African Way of Networking around Disability', *Disability & Society*, 26 (3): pp. 365–368

Moodley, R. and Bertrand, M. (2011) 'Spirits of a Drum Beat: African Caribbean Traditional Healers and Their Healing Practices in Toronto', *International Journal of Health Promotion and Education*, 49 (3): pp. 79–89

Morrison, E.E. (ed) (2009) *Health Care Ethics: Critical Issues for the 21st Century*. 2nd edn (Sudbury, MA: Jones & Bartlett)

Mukherjee, G. and Samanta, A. (2005) 'Wheelchair Charity: A Useless Benevolence in Community-Based Rehabilitation', *Disability & Rehabilitation*, 27 (10): pp. 591–596

Munyaradzi, M. (2012) 'Critical Reflections on the Principle of Beneficence in Medicine', *Pan-African Medical Journal*, 11, #29 [electronic document downloaded on 10 September 2012 from http://www.panafrican-med-journal.com/content/article/11/29/full].

Nagel, T. (1979) *Mortal Questions* (Cambridge: Cambridge University Press)

Nojhof, A., Wilderom, C. and Oost, M. (2012) 'Professional and Institutional Morality: Building Ethics Programmes on the Dual Loyalty of Academic Professionals', *Ethics and Education*, 7 (1): pp. 91–109

North, C.E. (2011) 'Embracing Honesty', *Teaching Education*, 20 (2): pp. 125–132

Nortvedt, P., Hem, M.H. and Skirbekk, H. (2011) 'The Ethics of Care: Role Obligation and Moderate Partiality in Health Care', *Nursing Ethics*, 18 (2): pp. 192–200

Nozick, R. (1974) *Anarchy, State and Utopia* (Oxford: Basil Blackwell)

Nussbaum, M. (2000) *Women and Human Development* (New York: Cambridge University Press)

Nussbaum, M. (2001) *Upheavals of Thought: The Intelligence of Emotions* (New York: Cambridge University Press)

Oakes, C.E. (2011) 'In Their Best Interest: The Challenge of Balancing Autonomy and Beneficence in Clinical Practice with Older Adults', *Gerontology Special Interest Section Quarterly*, 25 (9): pp. 1–4

Orme, J. (2002) 'Social Work: Gender, Care and Justice', *British Journal of Social Work*, 32 (6): pp. 799–814

Osmo, R. and Landau, R. (2006) 'The Role of Ethical Theories in Decision Making by Social Workers', *Social Work Education*, 25 (8): pp. 863–876

Paganini, M.C. and Yoshikawa Ergy, E. (2011) 'The Ethical Component of Professional Competence in Nursing', *Nursing Ethics*, 18 (4): pp. 571–582

Pascal, J. and Endacott, R. (2010) 'Ethical and Existential Challenges Associated with Cancer Diagnosis', *Journal of Medical Ethics*, 36 (5): pp. 279–283

Pavlish, C., Ho, A. and Rounkle, A.-M. (2012) 'Health and Human Rights Advocacy: Perspectives from a Rwandan Refugee Camp', *Nursing Ethics*, 19 (4): pp. 538–549

Peleg, R. (2008) 'Is Truth a Supreme Value?' *Journal of Medical Ethics*, 34 (5): pp. 325–326

Pellegrino, E.D. (2005) 'Some Things Ought Never to Be Done: Moral Absolutes in Clinical Ethics', *Theoretical Medicine and Bioethics*, 26 (6): pp. 469–486

Pellegrino, E.D. and Thomasma, D.C. (1988) *For the Patient's Good: The Restoration of Beneficence in Health Care* (New York: Oxford University Press)

Pellegrino, E.D. and Thomasma, D.C. (1993) *The Virtues in Medical Practice* (Oxford: Oxford University Press)

Rachels, J. (2010) *The Elements of Moral Philosophy*. 6th edn (New York: McGraw-Hill)

Rathburn, G. and Turner, N. (2012) 'Authenticity in Academic Development: The Myth of Neutrality', *International Journal for Academic Development*, 17 (3): pp. 231–242

Rawls, J. (1972) *A Theory of Justice* (Oxford: The Clarendon Press)

Reamer, F.G. (2006) *Social Work Values and Ethics*. 3rd edn (New York: Columbia University Press)

Reimer-Kirkham, S. (2009) 'Live Religion: Implications for Nursing Ethics', *Nursing Ethics*, 16 (4): pp. 406–417

Reisch, M. (2002) 'Defining Social Justice in a Socially Unjust World', *Families in Society: The Journal of Contemporary Social Services*, 83 (4): pp. 343–354

Ressler, A.B. (2006) 'An Existential Examination of Health Care Ethics', *International Journal for Human Caring*, 10 (1): pp. 61–67

Richard, C., Lajeunesse, Y. and Lussier, M. (2010) 'Therapeutic Privilege: Between the Ethics of Lying and the Practice of Truth', *Journal of Medical Ethics*, 36 (6): pp. 353–357

Richards, J.L. and Walker, R.N. (2011) 'Ninja Threats or Fantasy?' *Ethics & Behavior*, 21 (1): pp. 79–81

Ross, E. (2008) 'The Intersection of Cultural Practices and Ethics in a Rights Based Society: The Implications for South African Social Workers', *International Social Work*, 51 (3): pp. 384–395

Saldov, M. and Kakai, H. (2004) 'The Ethics of Medical Decision Making with Japanese-American Elders in Hawai'i: Signing Informed Consent Forms without Understanding Them', *Journal of Human Behavior in the Social Environment*, 10 (1): pp. 113–130

Scheyett, A., Kim, M., Swanson, J., Swartz, M., Elbogen, E., Van Dorn, R. and Ferron, J. (2009) 'Autonomy and the Use of Directive Intervention in the Treatment of Individuals with Serious Mental Illnesses', *Social Work in Mental Health*, 7 (4): pp. 283–306

Schroeder, D. (2010) 'Dignity: One, Two, Three, Four, Five, Still Counting', *Cambridge Quarterly of Healthcare Ethics*, 19 (1): pp. 118–125

Schwarz, S.H. (2007) 'Universalism Values and the Inclusiveness of our Moral Universe', *Journal of Cross-Cultural Psychology*, 38 (6): pp. 71–28

Sellman, D. (1996) 'Why Teach Ethics to Nurses?' *Nurse Education Today*, 16 (1): pp. 44–48

Sellman, D. (2009) 'Practical Wisdom in Health and social care: Teaching for Professional Phronesis', *Learning in Health and Social Care*, 8 (2): pp. 84–91

Sen, A. (1983) *Commodities and Capabilities* (Amsterdam: Elsevier)

Sercombe, H. (2010) *Youth Work Ethics* (London: Sage Publications)

Shaw, G.B. (1911) *The Doctor's Dilemma* (London: Constable)

Sheppard, M. (2002) 'Mental Health and Social Justice: Gender, Race and Psychological Consequences of Unfairness', *British Journal of Social Work*, 32 (6): pp. 779–797

Shun, K.-L. and Wong, D.B. (eds) (2004) *Confucian Ethics: A Comparative Study of Self, Autonomy and Community* (Cambridge: Cambridge University Press)

Simpson, C. (2002) 'Hope and Feminist Care Ethics: What Is the Connection?' *Canadian Journal of Nursing Research*, 34 (2): pp. 81–94

Singer, P. (1975) *Animal Liberation: A New Ethics for Our Treatment of Animals* (London: Jonathan Cape)

Singer, P. (2002) *One World: The Ethics of Globalization* (Melbourne: Text Publishing)

Smith, K.R. (20) 'Psychotherapy as Applied Science or Moral Praxis', *Journal of Theoretical and Philosophical Psychology*, 29 (1): pp. 34–46

Spence, D. and Smythe, L. (2007) 'Courage as Integral to Advancing Nursing Practice', *Nursing Praxis in New Zealand*, 23 (2): pp. 43–55

Starc, A. (2009) 'Nursing Professionalism in Slovenia: Knowledge, Power and Ethics', *Nursing Science Quarterly*, 22 (4): pp. 371–374

Stefkovitch, J. and O'Brien, M.G. (2004) 'Best Interests of the Student: An Ethical Model', *Journal of Educational Administration*, 42 (2): pp. 197–214

Steinberg, D. (2010) 'Altruism in Medicine: Its Definition, Nature, and Dilemmas', *Cambridge Quarterly of Healthcare Ethics*, 19 (2): pp. 249–257

Stevens, P. (2000) 'The Ethics of Being Ethical', *The Family Journal: Counseling and Therapy for Couples and Families*, 8 (2): pp. 177–178

Stocker, S.S. (2005) 'The Ethics of Mutuality and Feminist Relational Therapy', *Women and Therapy*, 28 (2): pp. 1–15

Straughair, C. (2012) 'Exploring Compassion: Implications for Contemporary Nursing. Part 1', *British Journal of Nursing*, 21 (3): pp. 160–164

Strike, K.A. and Soltis, J.F. (2004) *The Ethics of Teaching*. 4th edn (New York: Teachers' College Press)

Sykes, R.L. (2004) 'Ethical Attributes and Professional Skills Development', *The New Social Worker*, 11 (2): pp. 4–5

Tangwa, G.B. (2004) 'Between Universalism and Relativism: A Conceptual Exploration of the Problems in Formulating and Applying International Biomedical Ethics', *Journal of Medical Ethics*, 30 (1): pp. 63–67

Tesoriero, F. (2010) *Community Development* (French's Forest, NSW: Pearson Longman)

Thomas, B. (2008) 'Seeing and Being Seen: Courage and the Therapist in Cross-racial Treatment', *Psychoanalytic Social Work*, 15 (1): pp. 60–68

Thompson, R.J. (2011) 'Medical Futility: A Commonly Used and Potentially Abused Idea on Medical Ethics', *British Journal of Hospital Medicine*, 72 (2): pp. 969–969

Titmuss, R.M. (1971) *The Gift Relationship: From Human Blood to Social Policy* (New York: Pantheon Books)

Tronto, J. (1993) *Moral Boundaries: A Political Argument for an Ethics of Care* (New York: Routledge)

Tronto, J. (1998) 'An Ethic of Care', *Generations*, 22 (3): pp. 15–20

Trossman, S. (2011) 'Issues Up Close: The Practice of Ethics', *American Nurse Today*, 6 (11): pp. 32–33

Tsai, D.F. (2005) 'The Bioethical Principles and Confucius' Moral Philosophy', *Journal of Medical Ethics*, 31 (3): pp. 159–163

Tsang, (2008) 'Kairos and Practice Wisdom in Social Work Practice', *European Journal of Social Work*, 11 (2): pp. 131–143

Tschudin, V. (2003) *Ethics in Nursing: The Caring Relationship*. 3rd edn (Oxford: Butterworth-Heinemann)

Tupara, H. (2011) 'Ethics, Kawa and the Constitution: Transforming the System of Ethical Review in Aotearoa New Zealand', *Cambridge Quarterly of Healthcare Ethics*, 20 (3): pp. 367–379

Tutu, D. (1999) *No Future Without Forgiveness* (New York: Doubleday)

Uhrenfeldt, L. and Hall, E.O.C. (2007) 'Clinical Wisdom among Proficient Nurses', *Nursing Ethics*, 14 (3): pp. 397 398

United Nations (1948) *Universal Declaration of Human Rights* (New York: United Nations)

United Nations (2007) *Declaration on the Rights of Indigenous Peoples* (New York: United Nations)

van Hooft, S. (2011) 'Caring, Objectivity and Justice: An Integrative View', *Nursing Ethics*, 18 (2): pp. 149–160

Waghid, Y. and Smeyers, P. (2012) 'Reconsidering "ubuntu": On the Educational Potential of a Particular Ethic of Care', *Educational Philosophy and Theory*, 44 (Supplement 2): pp. 6–20

Walz, T. and Ritchie, H. (2000) 'Gandhian Principles in Social Work Practice: Ethics Revisited', *Social Work*, 45 (3): pp. 213–222

Weaver, H.N. (2002) 'Perspectives on Wellness: Journeys on the Red Road', *Journal of Sociology and Social Welfare*, 24 (1): pp. 5–15

Webb, S.A. (2009) 'Virtue Ethics' in M. Gray and S.A. Webb (eds), *Ethics and Value Perspectives in Social Work* (Basingstoke: Palgrave Macmillan)

Widdershoven, G., Abma, T. and Molewijk, B. (2009) 'Empirical Ethics as Dialogic Practice', *Bioethics*, 23 (4): pp. 236–248

Willette, C. (1998) 'Practical Discourse as Policy Making: An Application of Habermas' Discourse Ethics within a Community Mental Health Setting', *Canadian Journal of Community Mental Health*, 17 (2): pp. 27–38

Williams, B. (1981) *Moral Luck* (Oxford: Oxford University Press)

Wise, S. (1995) 'Feminist Ethics in Practice' in R. Hugman and D. Smith (eds), *Ethical Issues in Social Work* (London: Routledge)

Witz, A. (1992) *Professions and Patriarchy.* (London: Routledge)

Woodard, V. (1999) 'Achieving Moral Health Care: The Challenge of Patient Partiality', *Nursing Ethics*, 6 (5): pp. 390–398

World Federation of Occupational Therapy [WFOT] (2006) *Position Statement on Human Rights* (Forrestfield WA: WFOT)

World Medical Association [WMA] (1964) *Declaration of Helsinki*, as amended 2004 (Ferney-Voltaire: WMA)

World Medical Association [WMA] (2006) *International Medical Code of Ethics* (Ferney-Voltaire: WMA)

Yip, K. (2005) 'Chinese Concepts of Mental Health: Cultural Implications for Social Work Practice', *International Social Work*, 48 (4): pp. 391–407

Young, I.M. (1990) *Justice and the Politics of Difference* (Princeton, NJ: Princeton University Press)

Zomorodi, M. and Foley, B.J. (2009) 'The Nature of Advocacy vs. Paternalism in Nursing: Clarifying the "Thin Line"', *Journal of Advanced Nursing*, 65 (8): pp. 1746–1752

index